Barbara Pearlman's
SLENDERCISES

Barbara Pearlman

PHOTOGRAPHS BY GEORGE BENNETT

A DOLPHIN BOOK

Doubleday & Company, Inc., Garden City, New York   1980

DESIGNED BY MARILYN SCHULMAN

A DOLPHIN BOOK
Doubleday & Company, Inc.

ISBN: 0-385-15371-6

Library of Congress Catalog Card Number 79–7694

Copyright © 1980 by Barbara Pearlman

For Stephen and Aaron

Grateful acknowledgment to Lindy Hess, Carol Goldman, and Laura Van Wormer. Many thanks to Capezio Ballet Makers and Capezio East for their contributions to this book.

CONTENTS

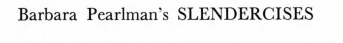

Barbara Pearlman's SLENDERCISES

1

Slendercises!

For the past eight years I have taught body conditioning (dance/exercise) to women of all shapes and sizes, ages and occupations. My private exercise service (house and office calls by appointment only) has taken me from the Greenwich Village brownstones of famous authors and actresses to the Eastside penthouses of television personalities. I've traveled from Wall Street conference rooms to Westside duplexes. One day I might be in the executive suite of a blue-chip company, the next in the apartment of a famous interior decorator. In many ways, I've been an exercise policewoman, keeping my clients on the slim and limber path.

Rarely, in my years of teaching, have I met a woman whose figure wasn't in need of some improvement. Most women need a bit of extra help in just one of those all-too-obvious problem spots. That's what this book is all about. There's a natural joy in looking one's best and it need not be a case of vanity. Within these pages you'll find problem-zone toners and short regimens to help *you,* personally, contour and redesign your body in order to achieve *your* most attractive shape. The plan is personalized, portable, quick, and, above all, easy to follow. The exercises will help you smooth out your unwanted lumps and bumps, making you appear trimmer even without losing weight. The reason they work is that when muscles are neglected (because of lack of activity) they foreshorten and fatty bulges form around them. As the muscles become strong and toned, the bulges disappear or at least become less obvious. Toned up muscles take up less room than flaccid, lazy ones. Thus you get a spot-reducing effect.

And if you're satisfied with your present shape, this book can help you keep the enviable shape you've worked so hard to achieve. Should you be among the satisfied few, remember, gravity is busy at work each minute of every day. Your buttocks, abdominals, upper arms, etc., are all susceptible to its ruthless tugging. It's up to you to fight that constant pull downward. The only way to challenge gravity is to keep your body toned and lifted through the proper trimming movements. By keeping your body toned and in good shape, you can look far younger than your actual years.

What exactly are your personal figure problems? Do you have a tendency to chubby thighs, flabby upper arms, oversized buttocks, or an incipient paunch? Whatever the flaw or flaws might be, there's no need to accept them as your permanent figure fate. Most problems can be considerably improved; some can be totally eliminated. While dieting can and does change your appearance by reducing those extra pounds, only exercise can "cure" your figure liabilities by remolding your shape to its correct and most attractive proportions. Think of exercise as the precision tool that can help you sculpture and redesign your body. Of course, this process can't and won't occur overnight. It probably took considerable time for your shape to arrive at its present condition and thus it will take time for you to tighten, tone, and redistribute. The key to your success must be dedication, enthusiasm, and a positive approach.

Should you also need to lose weight, find the appropriate diet for you—either on your own or, if necessary, with your physician's guidance. Determine how much weight you wish to lose in order to *realistically* satisfy your goals. Estimate sensibly, choosing a goal that is attainable, or you will inevitably become discouraged and give up. Remember, however, you must couple your diet with your personal shape-up plan. How many female dieters complain about losing weight from their bosom, for example, when the real problem spot continues to be their hips? Unfortunately, we are unable to determine where the weight drops from. That is not to say you should not diet to lose those unwanted pounds, but while doing so, pay close attention to your problem areas by practicing the exercises and regimens that will benefit you most. You will find the combination of both lines of attack will produce the results you are seeking.

Many of my clients find it particularly helpful to chart their personal progress by using what I call a "Shape-up—Slimber-up Chart." I've included one on page 10. Should you care to chart your own progress, make a point of recording your measurements (and your weight, if you wish) on the same day of every month. I guarantee you'll notice improvements if you're really consistent and practice the exercises that are best suited to your specific figure needs. With a bit of dedication and perseverance, your figure will change as the numbers diminish on your Shape-up—Slimber-up Chart.

To make the most of your slendercising plan, begin by taking a look at yourself—in the nude, of course—in a full-length mirror, from every angle. Only with every stitch of clothing removed can you assess your shape objectively and realistically. The mirror never lies! After you've given yourself a cold, calculating, honest appraisal, test yourself with some of the questions I've listed below:

— Is my present figure a help or hindrance in attaining my desires?
— Do I have one very obvious figure flaw? What is it?
— Where are my major problem spots? Between my shoulders and hips or from my hips down?
— Am I overweight? By how much?
— What specific improvement do I need?
— Is my bosom underdeveloped/too large/sagging?
— Are my upper arms flabby/weak/skinny?
— Is my waist fat/shapeless?
— Are my abdominals strong/weak/protruding?
— Are my hips flabby/too large/overweight?
— Are my buttocks firm/sagging/out of proportion/fat?
— Are my thighs fat/lacking tone?

These are just a sampling of the questions you might pose. Only after you've made an honest evaluation of your figure are you ready to select the toners and regimens suited to your personal needs and figure aspirations. The following list can serve as an over-all body guideline to strive for:

— Slender upper arms
— A well-developed bosom
— A slim waist
— Abdominals correctly flat for your body type
— Firm, shapely hips
— Firm, correctly proportioned buttocks
— Taut, sleek thighs

_2

Your Slimber-up Program

The slimber-up program in this book has been divided into three chapters. The first, Chapter 2, is devoted to exercise sets for the six most common figure problems: upper arms/bosom, waist, abdominals, hips, buttocks, and thighs. Each of these sets consists of ten supertoners placed in order of progressive difficulty. Chapter 3 consists of five individualized regimens, each incorporating two of the most common *combined* figure problems. Each of the regimens includes four exercises (two per area) and should take you no longer than five minutes to complete. Chapter 4 is a seven-minute Body Bonus. This is an easy-to-follow sequence designed to tone your muscles and improve your flexibility.

Ten Benefits You'll Derive from Your Slimber-up Program

— A more attractive, shapely figure

— Improved balance and coordination

— A more youthful-looking body

— Improved muscle tone

— Improved agility

— Increased flexibility

— Improved grace

— Improved circulation

— Increased energy

— Improved body alignment

— Practice the movements in a roomy, well-ventilated area (free of drafts) where physical and psychological distractions are at a minimum. If possible, try to practice in the same exercise "spot." In this way, your exercise space can become a special place in your daily life where you can comfortably retreat for several minutes and focus quietly on yourself. Do everything to insure peace, quiet, and privacy.

— Choose the time of day that works best for you. The same time each day is generally most effective since it gets you into the "exercise groove." Never exercise right after a heavy meal. Wait a minimum of forty-five minutes in order to eliminate the chance of nausea. Exercising too close to bedtime is also not recommended. It's too invigorating.

— Plan to devote at least fifteen minutes, five days a week, to your shape-up program. Try to exercise for the entire fifteen minutes without stopping. If you stop and start, you'll find your momentum and interest have lessened.

— Should you be unable to work on a carpeted surface and object to a bare floor, cover your practice surface with a large towel, mat, pad, or blanket. Make sure whatever you work on does not slip and slide while you move. (Instructions for making your own exercise mat can be found on page 8.)

— Your exercise attire should be comfortable and nonrestricting in order to allow you optimal flexibility. It should not bind you in any way. Remove eyeglasses, jewelry, and any confining or distracting paraphernalia.

— Do not rush through the movements, even if your time is limited. You are far better off doing six exercises correctly than sixteen improperly. Once you execute the first set of movements with ease and confidence, proceed to the next. Be certain to follow the instructions as closely as possible, giving full attention not only to the text but to the accompanying photographs. Fully comprehend what is required of you *before* you begin to move.

— Never strain in order to achieve an extreme position. When any part of your body is genuinely uncomfortable, that's a signal that you are applying yourself too strenuously. Let up a bit.

— Regardless of your age or shape, if you've had any serious medical condition or have had a severe accident, by all means consult your physician and discuss your intentions regarding your shape-up plan.

— Involve yourself and concentrate as you move. Be aware of the various parts of your body that are moving with each exercise. Understand which muscles control which movements. This will help you to perform the exercises correctly and will also increase and improve your over-all balance and coordination.

— A beginner will almost always experience some degree of muscle soreness when first starting an exercise program. The best way to ease the minor discomfort is to do some additional stretching. A warm bath can also give relief.

— It's far more pleasurable to exercise to music because of its encouraging and energizing effect. Disco and rock are favorites for many, since they have such an easy-to-follow beat and thus help to keep you moving in a fluid, rhythmic manner. It can be anything, however, from calypso to classic, depending on your mood and preference.

— Remember to BREATHE CORRECTLY! If you don't, you'll rob yourself of energy and diminish your ability to move with ease. In simplest terms, inhale (through your nose) when you lift, reach, stretch, or raise your body and limbs, and exhale (through your mouth) when you bend, release, relax, and bring your limbs close to your body. Let the breathing come as naturally as possible. (Breathlessness occurs when you hold too much air in and your lungs get so filled that you become uncomfortable.) When you exhale, do it fully, emptying your lungs totally.

— Generally, results can be seen (when you're serious and faithful about exercising) in approximately six to eight weeks' time. Keep in mind that the easiest areas to streamline are the waist and abdominals. The hips and thighs are next, followed by the upper arms and buttocks.

— Don't be overly critical or too tough on yourself. Advance at your own speed. Your present level of fitness will greatly determine how quickly you reach your figure goals. Allow your body to signal when it is ready to assume additional demands.

— Above all, stick with your program. The payoff in both physical and mental terms is worth far more than the effort. Make a pledge not to allow social, domestic, or business responsibilities to keep you from the exercise track. In fact, the busier you are and the more responsibilities you assume, the more important it is for you to be fit and slimber. There's simply no other way to keep in shape, even if the idea of exercising regularly for the rest of your life bores the leotards off of you. Keep this in mind when you feel your enthusiasm growing sluggish. No drugs, machines, or miracle beauty treatments can substitute for the real thing—your personal slimbering exercise routine.

How to Make Your Own Exercise Mat

Since standard exercise mats can be quite costly, why not whip up your own? It takes little effort or expense and works just fine. All you need are two large beach towels, identical in size, and a foam-rubber pad, which is available in various thicknesses at most department stores or sewing centers. The pad should be about one inch narrower and two inches shorter than the dimensions of the towels. Simply stitch the sides and one end of the towels together (use a sewing machine if one's available). Turn them inside out and insert the foam-rubber pad. Close the other end of the towels with snap fasteners (that way they can be easily laundered). Voilà! . . . you have an exercise mat.

Tape Up to Shape Up—Your Shape-up —Slimber-up Chart

Measure your progress on the same day of every month. Enter your present dimensions in the NOW column as well as the goals you wish to attain. Measure carefully (in the nude) according to the guidelines listed below. Be patient! Be optimistic! PERSEVERE!

UPPER ARMS — Three inches from the armpit.

BOSOM — Across the nipples. Be sure the tape is held level.

WAIST — At the narrowest part. Don't pull the tape too tight.

ABDOMINALS — At the bulge just below the navel.

HIPS I — At the largest curve.

HIPS II — At the side bulges and above the hips.

THIGHS — At the greatest bulge. Approximately three inches below the crotch.

It is now your job, once you've assessed your figure flaws, to choose, practice, and perfect those movements which will work best for you. Plan to devote approximately fifteen minutes, five days a week, to the toners which you need the most. Naturally, you may devote additional time if it is available. Never attempt, however, to practice too many exercises during one session. Instead, concentrate on performing only as many movements as you can realistically manage during the time you have allotted yourself. It is unwise to overload your practice session or to rush through the movements, substituting speed for thoroughness. The repetitions for each exercise are the *suggested* ones. You may of course decrease them if you have to or increase them gradually as your body becomes stronger and your endurance permits. It is not advisable, however, to increase the movements to more than double the indicated number. If you find yourself with time remaining before the fifteen minutes are completed, you may repeat one or several of the exercises. The time it will take you to perform your regimen will depend both on your ability as well as the tempo you establish.

Should you wish, for instance, to tone your upper arms as well as streamline your waistline, there will be twenty movements for you to practice. Naturally, you are not expected to perform all twenty exercises during one fifteen-minute session. In fact, no more than ten or twelve (at most) is recommended. The chart below illustrates how you might schedule yourself over a twenty-one-day period in order to obtain maximum benefits. After practicing all ten movements from both sets (upper arms and waist), you can mix and match the exercises for the remaining days. Because you will be able to create an endless variety of exercise sets, there should be no reason for boredom or monotony.

Shape-up—Slimber-up Chart

	NOW	MONTH 1	MONTH 2	MONTH 3	GOAL
UPPER ARMS					
BOSOM					
WAIST					
ABDOMINALS					
HIPS I					
HIPS II					
THIGHS					
WEIGHT					

Sample Schedule of Exercises for Shaping Up

	UPPER ARMS	WAIST
Day 1–3	1,2,3	1,2,3,4
Day 4–6	4,5,6,7	5,6,7,8
Day 7–9	8,9,10,2	9,10,1,3
Day 10–12	1,3,5,6	2,4,5,8
Day 13–15	6,9,1,8	8,7,10,3
Day 16–18	4,6,9	1,2,3,9,10
Day 19–21	3,5,8,1	2,4,5,8,9

The more figure flaws you wish to correct, the more exercises you have to choose from. In any case, make certain to include one exercise for each problem zone. This is preferable to working on a single figure flaw over a specific time period. It is recommended that you practice the toners of your choice for a three-day period before substituting others. This will assure familiarity with the movements, and thus you will be able to perform them with ease and effectiveness. You may, however, remain with the same exercises for longer than the recommended three days if you wish to. Remember, above all, you are not in competition with anyone. Work at your own speed, taking as long as necessary to familiarize yourself with the exercises. When your body has adapted to the exercise and you begin to attain flexibility and comfort with it, you will experience a wonderful sense of accomplishment. For some, this will come sooner than for others. If, for example, you are considerably out of shape and unaccustomed to exercising, you may wish to include only four or five exercises in each set for the first few weeks. That, too, is perfectly acceptable. On the other hand, the more advanced student will probably need less time to learn and perfect an exercise.

No matter what shape you're in, do not begin practicing additional movements until the ones you are working on have been perfected to the best of your ability. In general, for best results, spend approximately three days on each set of eight to ten movements. Once you have shaped up your problem zones, you may wish to work out an all-over shape-up regimen. This can be done by choosing at least one exercise from each of the six sets. Should time allow, you might also wish to include the seven-minute Body Bonus or several of the five-minute regimens.

Upper Arms/Bosom

Most exercises that help to correct flabby upper arms also aid in strengthening the pectorals (the supporting muscles which lie under the breasts). Thus, you are actually strengthening and toning both areas simultaneously. It is impossible to state categorically, however, that any system of exercise can change the size of the bosom or truly produce a desired effect on the breasts. That is because the bosom is not composed of muscle but of glands. These glands are embedded in fatty tissue. What you can do by strengthening the pectorals is make your bosom appear somewhat higher and firmer. That all-too-familiar schoolgirl chant, "I must, I must, I must increase my bust," accompanied by the correct exercise, can in fact give the bosom a more attractive appearance. Remember, the fringe benefits of almost any bosom exercise are more slender, shapely upper arms. As for other effective activities, swimming, yoga, tennis, and rowing are all beneficial for strengthening the pectorals and slimming the upper arms.

Are you somewhat buxom and unhappy about it? Then try to de-emphasize this feature as much as possible. Instead, play up one of your figure assets. Don't wear skin-tight sweaters or very revealing clothing, all of which draw attention to your bustline. You might instead adopt a looser, less clinging look. On the other hand, if you're as flat as a pancake, accept the fact that you'll never be a contender for the *Playboy* centerfold. Either make your flat chest into a fashion plus or play up another feature in order to detract attention from your bosom.

A woman who's been active and energetic all her life generally reaps the benefits. Her arms (the upper portions) are usually slender, smooth, and attractive without any sag underneath. If she's lost weight but hasn't exercised, she's probably plagued with loose, flabby skin under her arms. Fat has a tendency to form both on the inside and at the point where the arm joins the upper back. This fat is not only due to excess weight but due to muscle atrophy as well. Whereas men can camouflage their arms with jackets and shirts, a woman's alluring strapless dress won't camouflage hers. Because the tissues of the upper arm are so very delicate, it is imperative that constant attention (through exercise) be given this area.

Exercising in the water can be extremely beneficial for developing strength and tone in the upper arms and pectorals. Water movements bring into motion muscles in the under and back parts of the arm. The very fact that the water resists your movements makes each exercise even more effective and beneficial. The next time you have an opportunity to use a pool, try the following toner:

Bend your knees so that your shoulders are under water. Extend your arms in front with the palms facing out. Slowly push your arms apart until they are as far to the sides as possible. Then reverse your palms and bring your arms back together. This movement is similar to the breaststroke, which is also very effective as a bosom and upper-arm toner. Out of the water the arm motions of the backstroke can help to shape the upper arms. Make certain nothing is in your way. Then start one arm at a time, moving it up and back, making a wide circle as you go. As one arm reaches the top of the circle, start up and back with the other arm. The backstroke is more fun in the water, but works well on land too.

As another plus, exercises for the bosom and arms also tone the upper back and shoulder muscles which directly affect your posture. Did you realize the very appearance of your bosom is greatly affected by your postural habits? Naturally, if you permit your shoulders to round and your chest to sink in, your bosom is bound to sag more than if you stood or sat erectly. When you walk, try to be conscious of holding your head up and keeping your chest lifted. That does not mean you must carry yourself like a stiff, wooden soldier. Proper posture can and should be attained without force or strain. When you sit, do you tend to slouch and slump or do you hold yourself upright? When standing, do you try to maintain an erect spine? How about while driving? Do you collapse at the wheel? Remember, poor postural habits can truly play havoc with your figure, be it your hips, abdomen, bosom, or the rest of you.

In the morning or evening after you've showered or bathed, you might try this simple upper arm/bosom toner. Grasp your towel at both ends. With your arms extended high overhead, swing the towel back, keeping your arms totally straight and the towel taut. Repeat this exercise several times, gradually increasing the number of repetitions. A definite tug at the front of your shoulders indicates a need for strengthening your shoulder muscles as well. I generally try to do ten or twelve of these towel toners once or twice a day. Give them a try; they're really effective.

Another at home upper arm/bosom exercise can be done right in your kitchen while you await the coffee to perk or the soufflé to rise. Take two unopened soup cans (or cans of comparable size) and use them for weights. Extend your arms out to the sides until they are totally straight. Form large circular motions backward ten times, then forward ten times. You can also do this exercise with your arms extended upward.

While watching television, why not try another easy shaper. Bend your right arm at the elbow so that the hand touches the center of your upper back. Your elbow should be pointed straight up. Next bend your left arm placing the back of your left hand against your lower spine. Carefully work your right hand down as you simultaneously inch your left hand up. Try to make your hands meet so that the fingers of each hand clasp one another. Hold this position for about ten seconds. While doing this movement, move your hands very slowly, keeping the upright elbow as raised as possible. Not only will this exercise do wonders for your upper arms and bosom, but it will strengthen your back and improve your posture as well. It's also ideal for giving those seldom exercised muscles around and under your shoulder blades a chance to develop. In addition, many of my clients find this movement can be extremely beneficial for relieving tension in the center of the back and the shoulders.

UPPER ARMS/BOSOM 1

PLACEMENT: Sit with your ankles crossed. Extend your arms overhead.

MOVEMENT: Alternating arms, reach upward eight times. Round your back and place your palms on the floor. Bounce up and down four times. Uncurl slowly to the original position.

TOTAL REPETITION: Four times.

Keep your chin slightly lifted as you reach upward.

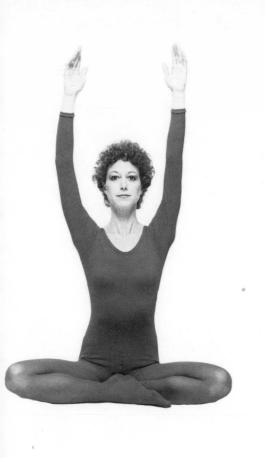

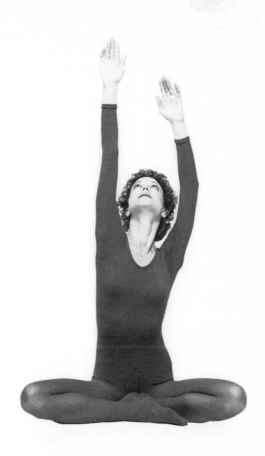

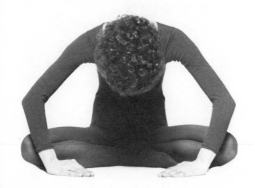

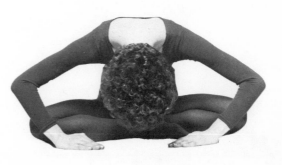

PLACEMENT: Lie flat with your knees bent and your feet parallel on the floor. Rest your arms at your sides, palms down.

MOVEMENT: Stretch your arms overhead until they touch the floor, palms up. Hold for three counts. Lower your arms to the original position as you press your spine against the floor.

TOTAL REPETITION: Ten times.

As you stretch your arms overhead, your rib cage will lift somewhat. This exercise not only tones the arms and pectorals, but also strengthens the back.

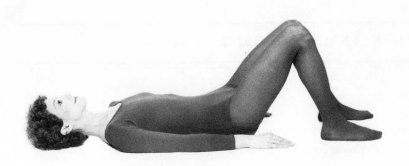

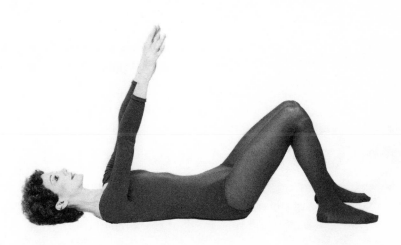

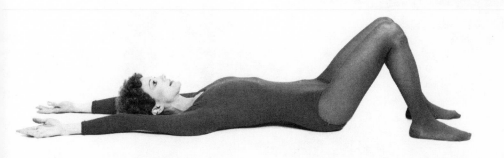

PLACEMENT: Sit with your ankles crossed and your hands clasped behind your head. Open your elbows to the sides.

MOVEMENT: Keeping your hands laced together, straighten your arms upward, palms facing up. Hold for two counts, then release.

TOTAL REPETITION: Twelve times.

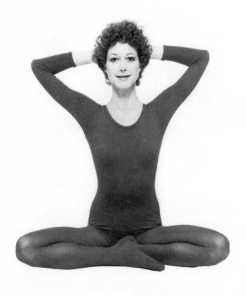

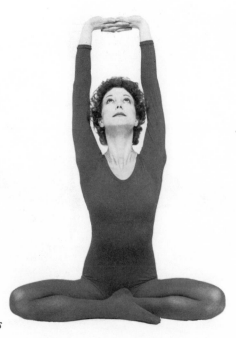

UPPER ARMS/BOSOM 4

PLACEMENT: Sit with your ankles crossed. Place your hands on your waist.

MOVEMENT: Round your back and lower your head. Allow your elbows to release forward. Hold for two counts. Lift to a straight-back position, pulling your elbows as far back as possible.

TOTAL REPETITION: Eight times.

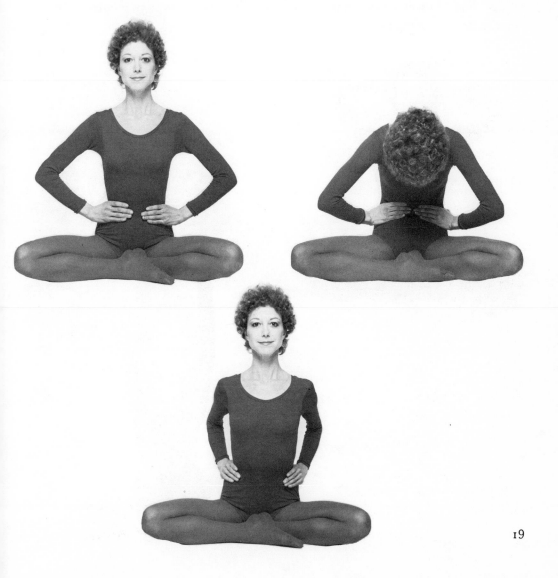

UPPER ARMS/BOSOM 5

PLACEMENT: Stand with your feet wide apart and parallel. Clasp your hands behind your body.

MOVEMENT: Twist your upper body to the left. At the same time raise your arms. Bounce them upward three times. Return center, lower your arms, and repeat, twisting to the right.

TOTAL REPETITION: Five times for each side.

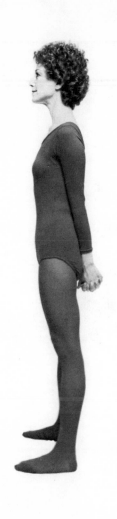

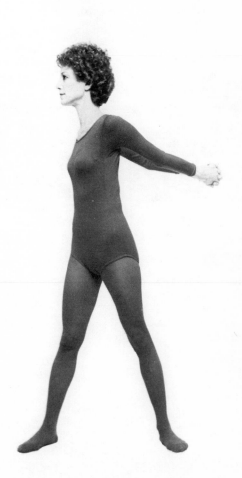

PLACEMENT: Sit with your ankles crossed, back erect. Clasp your hands behind your head, elbows open to the sides.

MOVEMENT: Round your back and lower your head as close to the floor as possible. At the same time, bring your elbows together. Hold for three counts. Lift your head and body slowly, opening the elbows as you straighten your back.

TOTAL REPETITION: Ten times.

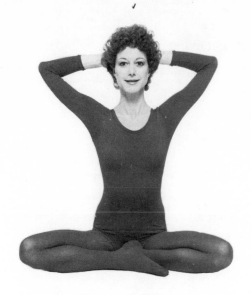

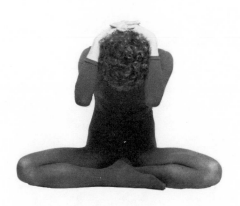

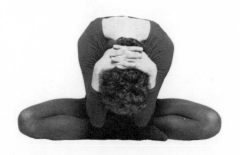

PLACEMENT: Sit with your knees out and the soles of your feet together. Rest your hands on your toes.

MOVEMENT: Stretch upward with your right arm. Reach forward, stretching as far as possible. Next lift your arm and body until your back is straight. Lower the arm and repeat with the left arm.

TOTAL REPETITION: Six times for each side.

As you reach forward, press your knees down and keep your buttocks stationary.

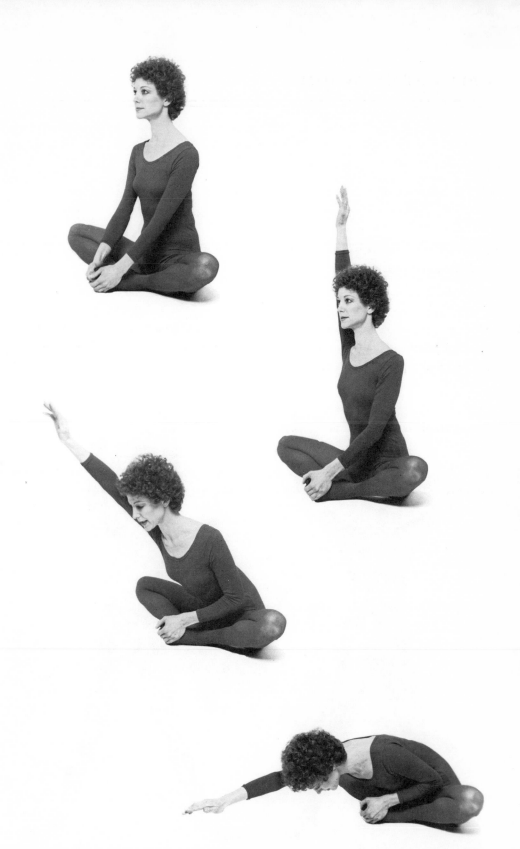

PLACEMENT: Stand with your feet wide apart and slightly turned out. Lace your hands behind your head, elbows open to the sides.

MOVEMENT: Stretch your arms upward until they are straight, palms up. Tilt from the waist to the right, then to the left. Return center before lowering the arms to the original position.

TOTAL REPETITION: Ten times.

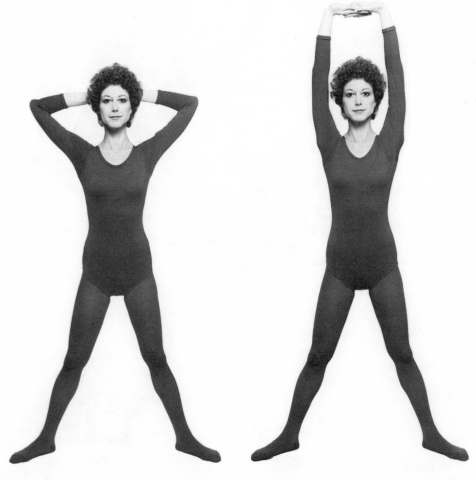

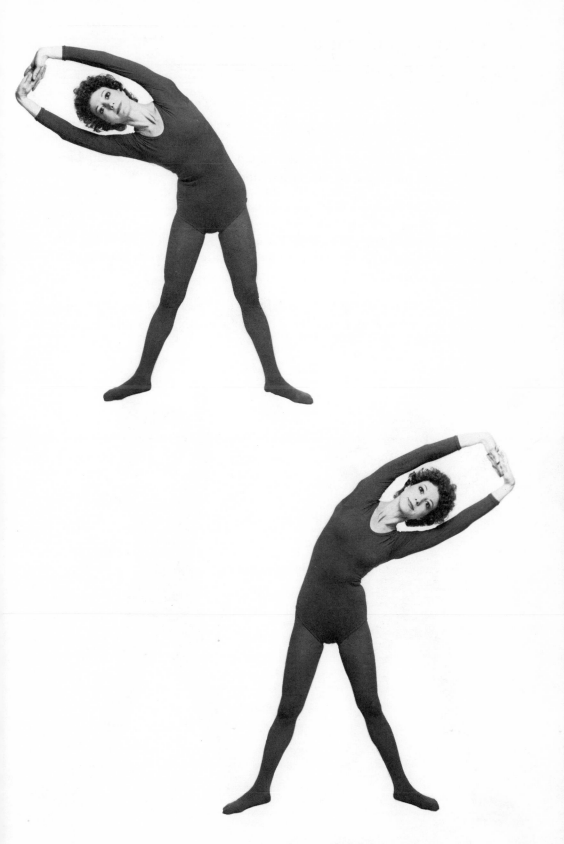

PLACEMENT: Stand with your feet wide apart and parallel. Extend your arms overhead, fingers interlaced.

MOVEMENT: Release your body forward, from the hips. Round your back and swing your arms between your legs. Then swing forward, lifting to the starting position.

TOTAL REPETITION: Ten times.

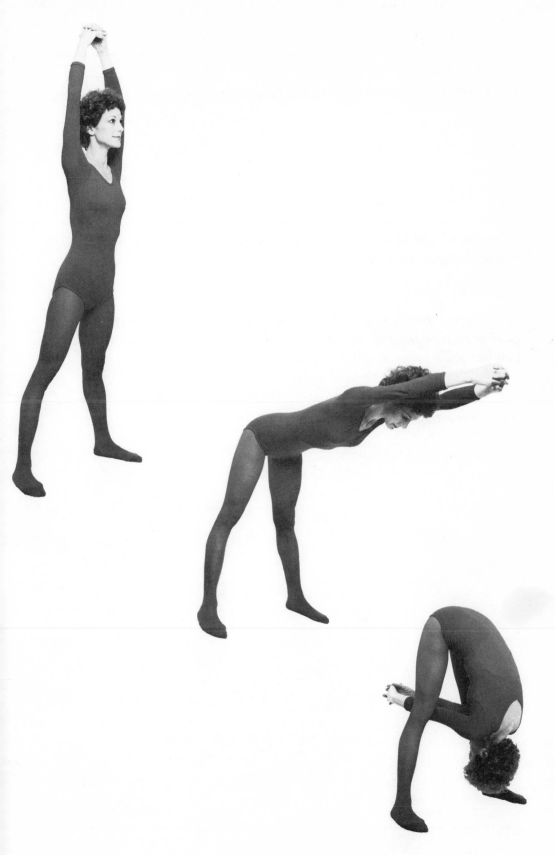

PLACEMENT: Sit with your legs extended to the sides. Clasp your hands behind your body, fingers interlaced.

MOVEMENT: Round your back and lower your head as close to the floor as possible. At the same time, lift your arms. Hold for three counts. Lift your body back to position as you lower your arms.

TOTAL REPETITION: Ten times.

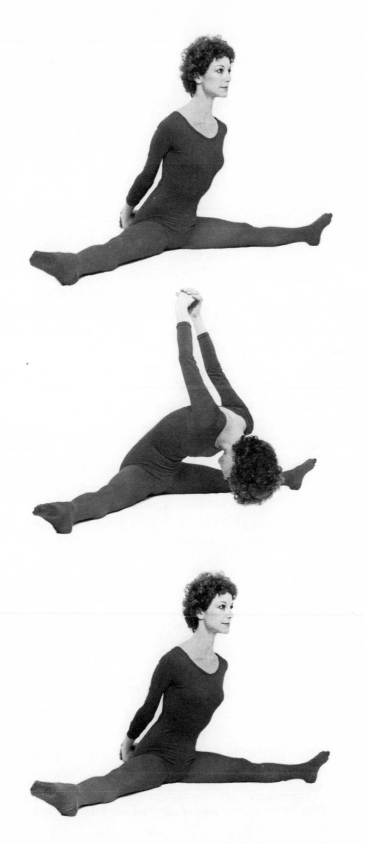

Waist

The natural shape for a woman's body to be is narrower in the waist than directly above or below. It should look more like an hourglass than a box. When this narrowness begins to disappear a woman can almost always be certain she's on the way to "expanding." When posture is neglected as well, the upper body slips downward, obliterating the waistline and adding weight to the lower body. Not only does this ruin the line of the waist, but it places an increased burden on the legs. Improper posture can truly throw the entire body out of line, causing endless problems.

The most effective waistline whittlers are those exercises which create a lift in the torso area. By stretching in the correct manner, with the right movements, one can actually stimulate muscle tone, which in turn helps to keep the upper body strong, lifted, and erect. The waistline also responds well to movements that encourage bending and twisting. It is through the regular practice of these sorts of movements that a woman can reproportion her body and attain a more hourglass shape. As you increase activity and stimulate circulation in the waist area, you'll eventually notice significant changes in your dimensions.

Side stretches such as the movements on page 49 are very beneficial. For best results when practicing any side movements, remember to keep the palm of your raised hand facing upward. This little trick produces a greater stretch all the way past your waist to your hips. One of my favorite waist whittlers is illustrated on page 35. This exercise can be done while standing or while lying down. Should you practice it lying flat on the floor, think of yourself as a rubber band being stretched from fingertips to toes on alternate sides of your body. I particularly enjoy doing this stretch in bed in the morning. I know it's not only slenderizing my waist but it's also great for eliminating stiffness after a night's sleep. One hint to keep in mind as you practice this exercise: inhale as you stretch, hold the stretch for a count of two, then exhale on the release.

Stretches done on the floor with your legs extended to the sides (see page 49) are also extremely effective for minimizing the waist. As you practice these side stretches, let the movement start at the torso, not with the arms or head. Also remember to keep that palm facing upward. Finally, with all side stretches executed on the floor, be certain to keep your buttocks stationary. If you allow them to lift off the floor, you will lessen the beneficial aspect of this sort of movement.

Consider yourself fortunate if your waistline is your only figure flaw. It's just about the easiest part of your body to slenderize. It's also the area that seems to show signs of change (for the better as well as the worse) the fastest. You will discover that once you've lost an inch or two in your waist, your entire body will have a more attractive, youthful appearance. Many of my clients who are a bit too curvy and have problems reducing other parts of their body (thighs, buttocks, upper arms, etc.) appear years younger as soon as they reduce those excess inches in their waistline. Remember, too, that at the same time you're slimming and trimming your waistline, you will be strengthening your abdominals and back muscles. In fact, many exercises for almost any other part of your figure will simultaneously benefit your waist as well.

I usually try to encourage my clients to use everyday situations to their best advantage. Twist and turn when looking for something, bend and stretch when reaching for an object. Make every attempt to use your body to its fullest range of motion whenever the opportunity presents itself, since no fat can remain in a place that is constantly being twisted and bent, stretched and lifted. You might also consider keeping some important figure tips in mind in order to best camouflage a not-so-terrific waistline. Wear narrow belts and monotone colors, and do try to keep details and trimmings away from the waistline. Bright colors near the waist should also be avoided.

PLACEMENT: Lie on your back with your legs extended in front and your arms relaxed at your sides.

MOVEMENT: Slowly stretch your right arm overhead as you simultaneously flex* your right foot. Hold for two counts, then release, and repeat with the left arm and foot.

TOTAL REPETITION: Six times for each side.

As you stretch, think of your body as a rubber band being pulled in two directions.

---

* Flex: This refers to the position of your feet. When you flex your foot, the toes are pulled back toward your leg and the heel is pressed forward. Flexing is the opposite of pointing, which is when the toes are pushed forward and downward.

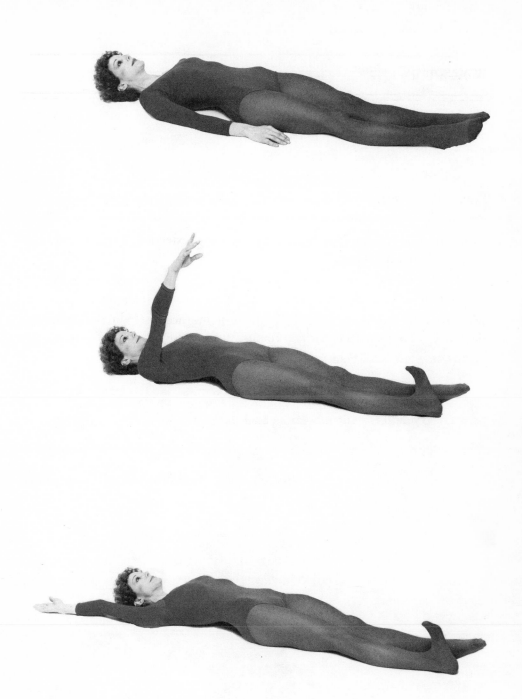

PLACEMENT: Stand with your feet wide apart. Clasp your hands together at chest level, arms straight.

MOVEMENT: Swing your upper body to the right. In this position, twist further right three times. Return to center and repeat, twisting to the left.

TOTAL REPETITION: Four times for each side.

Try to keep your feet stationary throughout this movement.

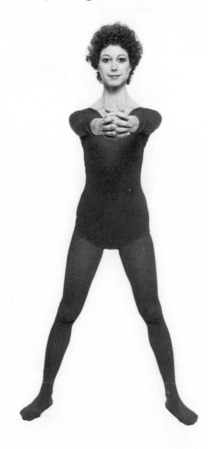

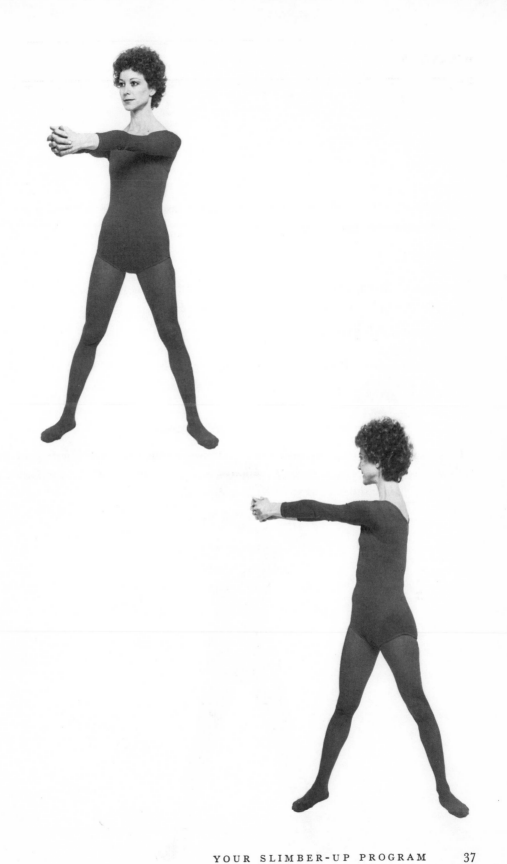

PLACEMENT: Sit with your ankles crossed. Extend your arms to the sides at shoulder level.

MOVEMENT: Keeping your lower body stationary, isolate your torso by stretching from side to side.

TOTAL REPETITION: Twenty times.

This exercise takes a bit of concentration. Imagine that you have a string attached to each side of your rib cage, pulling you from right to left. Press the opposite buttock into the floor as you stretch to other side.

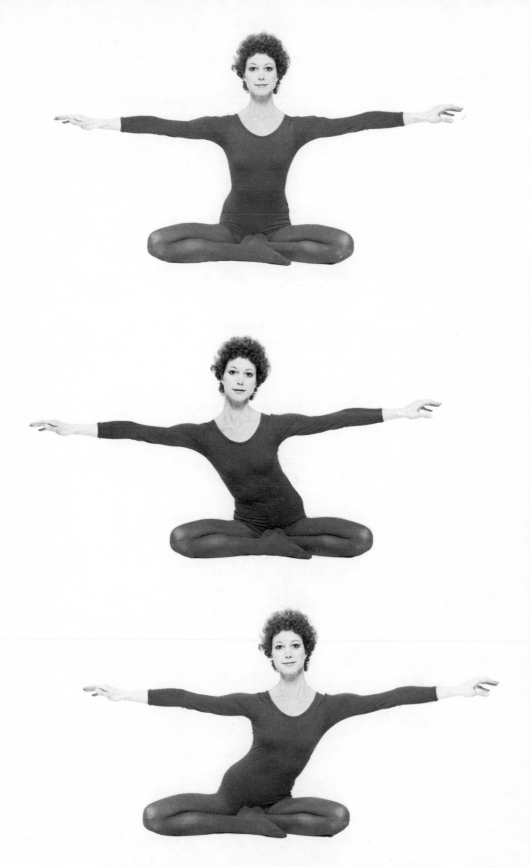

PLACEMENT: Sit with your ankles crossed. Rest your hands on the floor near your knee and twist your upper body to the right.

MOVEMENT: Bounce up and down four times. Try to lower your left cheek as close to your right knee as possible. Swing to the left and repeat, lowering your right cheek to your left knee.

TOTAL REPETITION: Three times for each side.

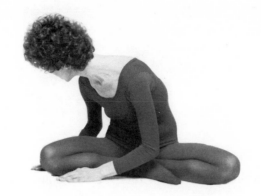

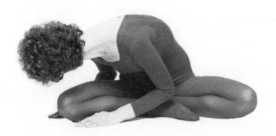

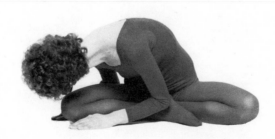

PLACEMENT: Sit with your legs extended as far to the sides as possible. Twist your upper body to the right. Extend your arms in front of your body at chest level.

MOVEMENT: Stretch forward from your waist. Then pull all the way back. Repeat this forward and back motion four times. Twist to the left and repeat.

TOTAL REPETITION: Three times for each side.

It is important that you keep your buttocks stationary on the forward-stretching motion.

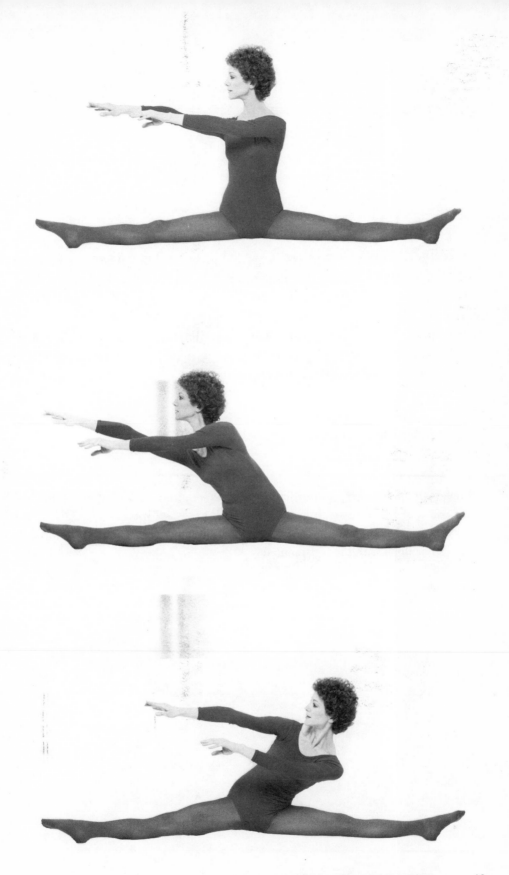

PLACEMENT: Sit with your legs extended as far to the sides as possible, feet flexed. Place your hands on your hips.

MOVEMENT: Lean to the right. Slide your right hand toward your right foot. Lower the side of your head as close to your right leg as possible. Hold the stretch for three counts. Repeat, leaning to the left.

TOTAL REPETITION: Five times for each side.

When leaning to either right or left, press your opposite buttock down. This will give you a maximum stretch in your waist. If you wish, you can also do this exercise with three bounces instead of sustaining the stretch. Try it both ways. It can also be done with the toes pointed.

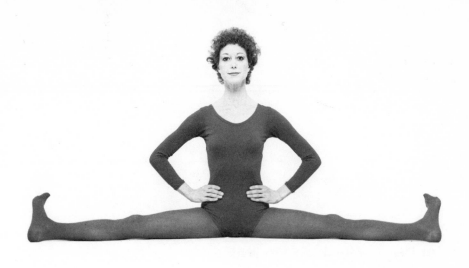

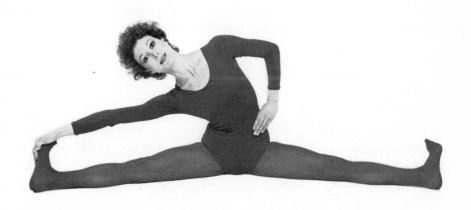

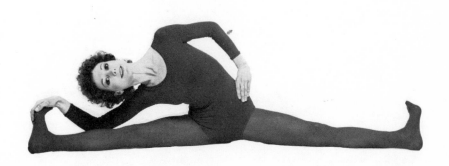

PLACEMENT: Sit with your knees bent and your back rounded. Rest only your toes on the floor. Extend your arms in front.

MOVEMENT: Slide your feet on the floor until your legs are straight. At the same time, straighten your back and extend your arms upward. Then slide your feet back into place, lower your arms, and resume the original rounded back position.

TOTAL REPETITION: Twelve times.

This movement can be done at a fairly rapid tempo.

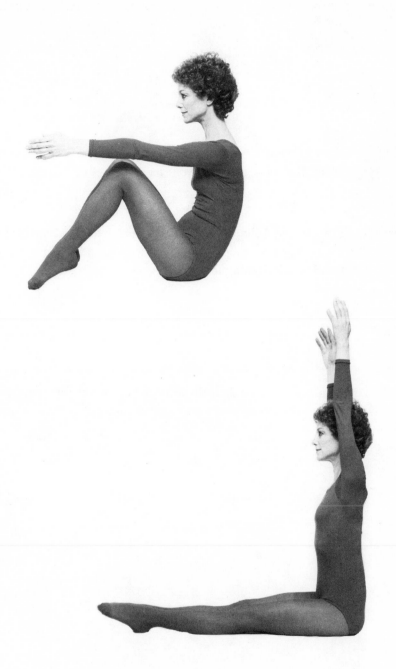

PLACEMENT: Sit with your legs extended to the sides, knees bent and soles of your feet on the floor. Rest your hands on your legs.

MOVEMENT: Lean to the right. Slide your right hand toward your right foot as your left arm arches overhead, palm up. Bounce up and down three times. Return to center and repeat, leaning to the left.

TOTAL REPETITION: Six times for each side.

This movement can also be done as a single stretch, without the bounce. After completion of this exercise, bring your legs together and gently bounce them up and down several times.

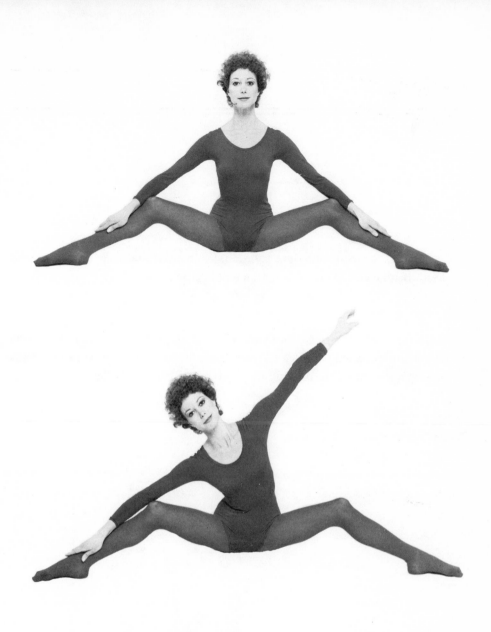

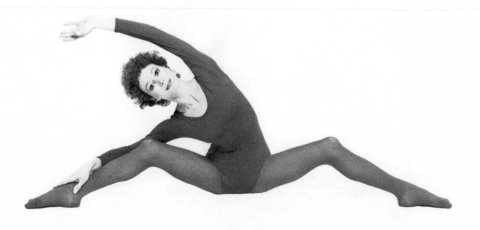

PLACEMENT: Sit with your right leg extended in front and your arms extended overhead. Bend your left leg and rest the foot near your left buttock.

MOVEMENT: Slowly stretch forward from your hips, lowering your torso and arms over the extended right leg. Stretch forward, then lift your torso and arms to the original position. Repeat six times. Repeat with the left leg in front.

TOTAL REPETITION: Two times for each leg.

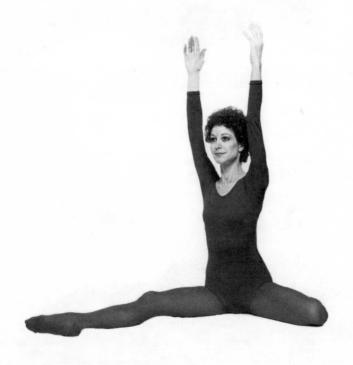

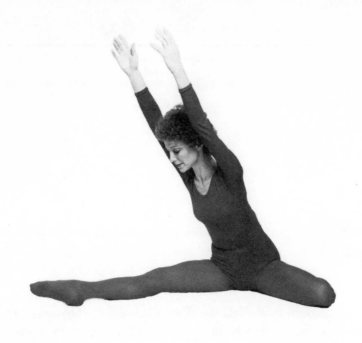

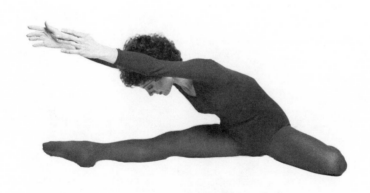

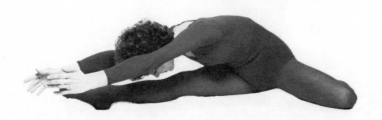

PLACEMENT: Sit with your legs extended to the sides, toes pointed. Clasp your hands over your head.

MOVEMENT: Twist your torso to the left. Lean forward and lower your body over the leg. Hold for two counts. Slowly lift, twist to center, and repeat, twisting to the right.

TOTAL REPETITION: Six times for each side.

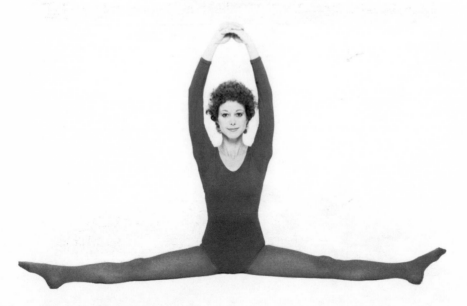

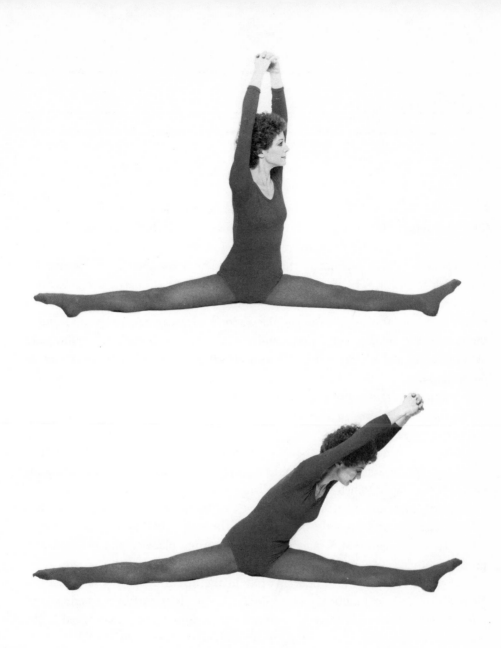

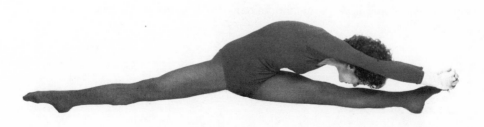

Abdominals

The abdominals form a muscular corset three layers thick between the diaphragm and the pelvis. They are responsible for bending the trunk from side to side, rotating it, and supporting the stomach. The abdominal structure permits expansion to occur. The more one eats and bloats the stomach, the larger the area becomes. This naturally has an all-too-obvious negative effect on one's health and appearance. The longer the abdominal area remains overexpanded, the greater the chance that the abdominal wall will lose its tone. Therefore, one of the first rules of abdominal health and beauty is not to allow the abdomen to overexpand.

Softness, sagging, protrusion, and general overweight are the most common problems relating to the abdomen. Fortunately, problems with this area are not impossible to correct. The abdomen responds well to the proper toning exercises. This is not to imply that these problems are to be regarded lightly. Deterioration of the abdomen often reflects grave danger to one's health and well-being. When the abdomen protrudes because the wall has lost its muscle tone, the internal organs that are held in place by the abdominal muscles become misplaced. They in turn sag with the sagging of the wall. This can be a serious condition since an organ that is sagging out of its normal place cannot function in a proper manner.

Posture, too, plays an important role in the appearance of your abdomen. Your abdominals will naturally protrude if you slouch or carry your body out of line. When posture is incorrect, some muscle groups become shortened while others stretch unnaturally in order to accommodate the situation. All-over fatigue is another by-product of weak abdominals. When the abdominals can't do their share in supporting the body, overworked muscles responsible for other jobs simply can't cope with the extra burden and fatigue results.

In order to maintain correct alignment, you must stretch the proper muscle groups. It may simply be a matter of strengthening certain areas which over the years have become lazy (your abdominals, for instance). To best visualize correct alignment, with your abdominals properly placed, think of your body as a string of pearls, one atop the other. All the pearls will fall out of line if the string is slack. When the string is firmly held, the pearls remain correctly placed. In addition, good posture can actually conceal figure flaws, whereas bad posture only accentuates them.

Diet alone cannot improve the condition of your abdominals. Many clients begin lessons with me after having lost significant amounts of weight. Often their abdominals still protrude in spite of the weight loss. One of my clients, a young, aspiring model hardly tipped the scale at one hundred pounds, yet she had an actual "pot." That was because her abdominals totally lacked tone. Being slender is no insurance; in fact, it can make a tummy appear all the more unsightly. Within two months' time, practicing the proper strengthening movements, her belly had diminished considerably.

I do not wish to imply, however, that a slight feminine curvature is unattractive or abnormal. In many cases, because of a woman's bone structure and build, a curvature within bounds is both acceptable and attractive. The flat tummy obsession which is so important to many women is often both impossible and unnecessary to achieve. Some women are naturally curvaceous, with full hips and full bosoms. Such women will tend to have slight curvatures of the abdomen, even if their weight is right on target. In such a case, it would be decidedly unnatural and unrealistic to attempt to firm the abdomen to the flattened state of a pancake. What I'm saying, in short, is that you should strive only to attain the best, most attractive physical condition possible for your basic body structure.

Many women feel they can hide the poor state of their abdomen by flattening it with a girdle or corset. Since these constricting garments limit the use of the abdominals, the potbellied condition becomes more severe and pronounced. What one should do instead is develop one's natural girdle of muscle, not rely on undergarments for support.

For genuine tone and strength of the abdominal area, you must exercise the muscles regularly and correctly. Remember, too, *you need not agonize to exercise correctly.* For example, many women do harm to their back by practicing what they believe is an effective abdominal toner. They lie flat on the floor and lift or lower both legs simultaneously. Because it hurts, they believe they're doing themselves a good turn. Nothing could be further from the truth. Lifting and lowering both legs at the same time is known to cause all sorts of problems. The reason is that most women are unable to lift or lower their legs without arching their backs or lifting their rib cages. Unless this particular movement is executed with the spine totally flat against the floor, and the abdominals properly contracted, it can be harmful. By arching the back, you place extreme pressure on the lower spine and thus invite injury. In short, refrain from this exercise even if you've been told (or think) it does wonders for your abdominals.

One abdominal exercise that I do recommend can be done just about anytime or anywhere. It's a simple contraction. During the day as you sit, stand, move, and work, you can exercise your abdominals simply by pulling them in. Try it while you wait in line at the movies or at the supermarket check-out counter. Just pull your abdomen in (but don't hold your breath) and maintain the contraction for the count of five. Then release slowly. It's an easy drill, but one that can help you become more aware of your abdominal muscles as you simultaneously strengthen them. Once you really get into the habit, your abdominals will begin to work for you.

While exercising with any of the movements in this book, be conscious of holding your abdominals in. For example, turn to page 27. As you stand, tilting your upper body from side to side, the tendency will be to allow your abdominals to relax and so to protrude. Be aware of this as you exercise, especially with lateral movements. On page 63 you will find an exercise that requires you to release your upper body halfway back to the floor as illustrated in the photo. In any movement of this sort, be certain that you do not go back too far. If you do, you will reduce its effectiveness. In such an exercise, try to hold the contraction at the point of maximum stress. The same holds true for sitting-up exercises. If you sit up all the way until your back is totally erect, you decrease the benefit of the movement. Again, become aware of the point of optimal stress and stop there.

Finally, should you be a victim of lower-back aches and pains, weak abdominals are more often than not the real culprits. That's why pregnancy is such a test for the strength of a woman's abdominals. She will rarely complain of lower-back pains if her abdominals are strong and elastic. When, on the other hand, tone is poor and the muscles weak, not only can a pregnant woman's appearance and posture be grossly unattractive, but a severe and annoying backache can also become her constant companion. A protruding potbelly generally indicates weak abdominals. Weak abdominals mean that your body must be improperly aligned. A body out of line inevitably leads to fatigue and lower-back pain. Correcting this condition will not only improve your overall appearance (pregnant or not), but will also help you keep your back strong and healthy. Should your back already be giving out pain signals and your belly protruding, start to improve this condition today by strengthening your abdominals with the following set of exercises.

PLACEMENT: Sit with your knees bent. Place the soles of your feet parallel and about twelve inches apart. Extend your arms in front at chest level.

MOVEMENT: Release your body halfway back. At the same time, slide your left leg forward until it is straight. Hold for two counts. Resume the original position and repeat with your right leg. Repeat ten times. Then extend both legs in front, round your back, and rest your hands on your ankles. Bounce up and down four times.

TOTAL REPETITION: Two times.

Remember not to release your body too far back. Stop at the point when you are supported by your lower spine.

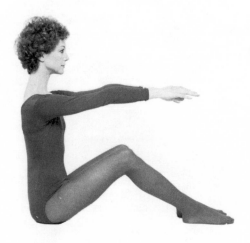

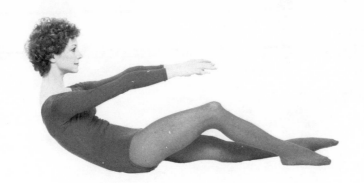

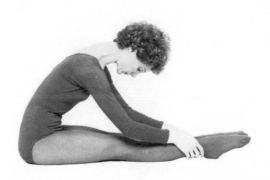

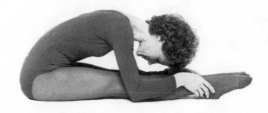

PLACEMENT: Lie on your back, knees bent close to your chest. Rest your arms at your sides.·

MOVEMENT: Keeping the left knee in place, extend your right leg until it is straight and several inches off of the floor. Hold for three counts. Bring the leg back into position and repeat with the left leg. Repeat eight times. Draw your knees to your chest and rock them forward and back four times.

TOTAL REPETITION: Two times.

As you extend the leg forward, make certain that your abdominals are contracted.

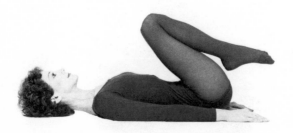

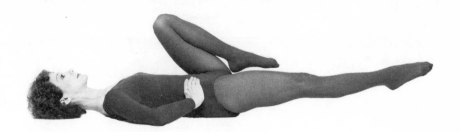

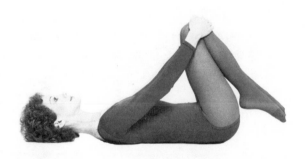

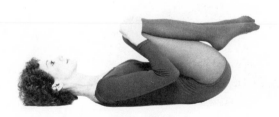

PLACEMENT: Sit with your legs extended in front, back erect. Clasp your hands in front at chest level.

MOVEMENT: Release your upper body forward, from the hips, as far as possible. Then contract back until your lower spine rests on the floor. This forward and back motion can be done fairly rapidly.

TOTAL REPETITION: Twenty times.

This exercise is similar to a rowing motion. Remember to contract your buttock and abdominal muscles as you release back. This will help you maintain better control.

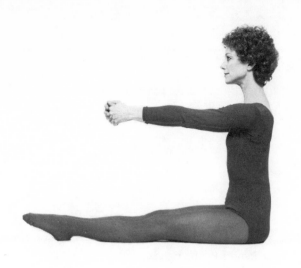

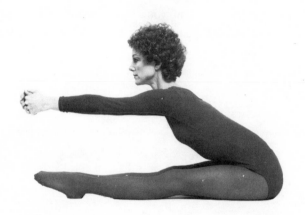

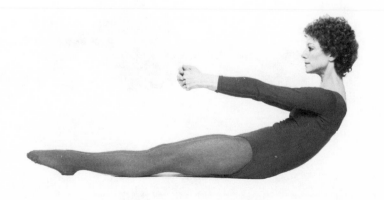

PLACEMENT: Lie on your back with your knees close to your chest. Interlace your fingers and rest your head in your hands.

MOVEMENT: Lift your upper body (head, neck, and shoulders) off the floor as you bring your elbows together. Extend your legs upward. Then bend them. Finally lower your body and release your elbows to the original position. The count is: lift—extend—bend—release.

TOTAL REPETITION: Ten times.

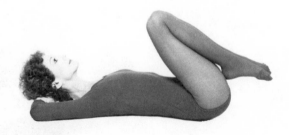

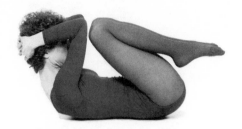

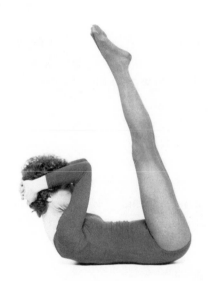

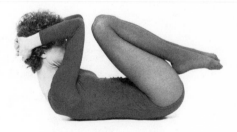

PLACEMENT: Lie on the floor with your right leg extended in front. Rest your left foot on the floor. Extend your arms on the floor over your head.

MOVEMENT: Lift your head, neck, and shoulders off the floor. Simultaneously swing your arms forward. Hold for two counts, then slowly release. Repeat four times with the right leg, then four times with the left.

TOTAL REPETITION: Three times.

Try to maintain the contraction at the maximum stress point. Do not sit up all the way. Stop when your middle back is no longer resting on the floor.

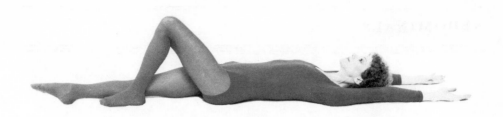

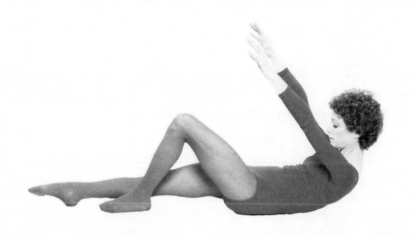

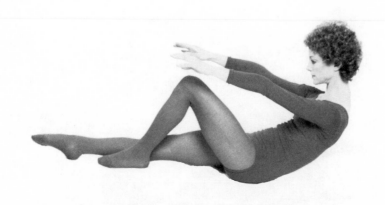

PLACEMENT: Lie on your back, knees close to your chest. Rest your arms at your sides.

MOVEMENT: Extend your right leg forward. Lift the leg as high as possible. Lower it practically to the floor before bending it to the original position. The count is: extend—lift—lower—bend. Repeat with the left leg.

TOTAL REPETITION: Six times for each leg.

When extending the leg forward, keep it several inches off of the floor.

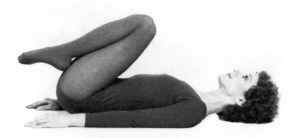

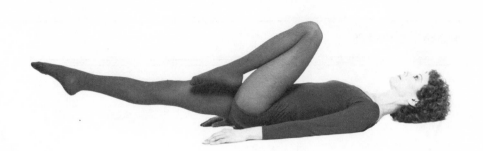

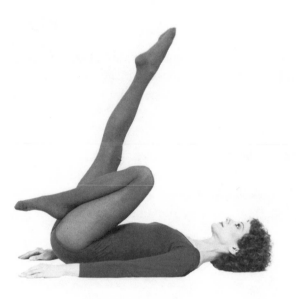

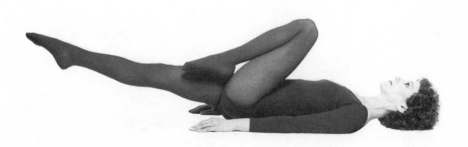

PLACEMENT: Lie on your back with your legs extended straight upward. Rest your arms on the floor.

MOVEMENT: Keeping your abdominals contracted, slowly lower your right leg until it is approximately ten inches from the floor. Lift the leg and repeat with the left leg.

TOTAL REPETITION: Six times for each leg.

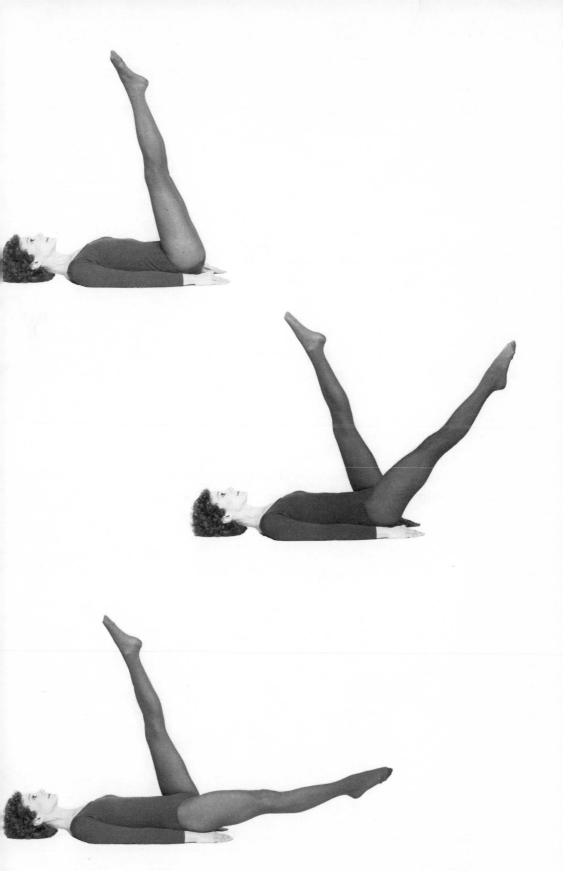

ABDOMINALS 8

PLACEMENT: Lie on your back with your knees bent close to your chest. Rest your hands on your waist.

MOVEMENT: Extend your left leg forward until it is straight and several inches off of the floor. Bounce the leg up and down six times, touching the floor each time. Bend the knee and repeat with the right leg.

TOTAL REPETITION: Four times for each leg.

Do not lift the leg any higher than illustrated in the photograph.

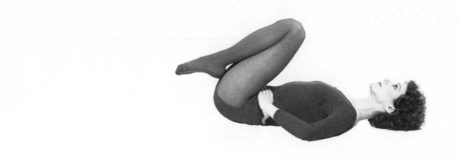

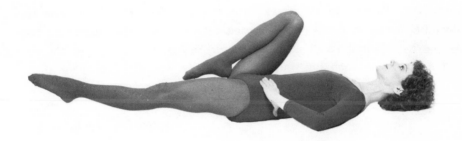

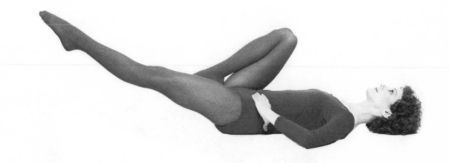

PLACEMENT: Lie on your back, legs extended in front. Rest your arms on the floor over your head.

MOVEMENT: Roll up to a halfway sit-up position with your knees bent, toes pointed and resting on the floor. Your back should be rounded. As you lift your body, your arms will naturally swing forward. Next, slide your legs on the floor and simultaneously reach for your ankles. Finally, uncurl slowly back to the floor. The count is: lift—stretch—uncurl.

TOTAL REPETITION: Ten times.

Try to keep this movement fluid and controlled. As you release back to the floor, contract your abdominal and buttock muscles.

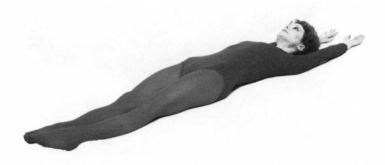

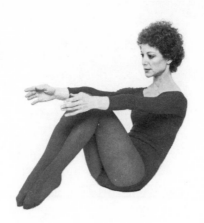

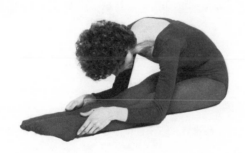

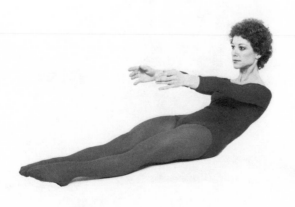

PLACEMENT: Sit with your legs extended to the sides. Clasp your hands over your head.

MOVEMENT: Slowly tilt your body from left to right. Repeat eight times. Next, round your back, lower your head, and place your palms on the floor. Bounce up and down four times.

TOTAL REPETITION: Three times.

On the tilting motion, make certain to stretch upward each time you return to center.

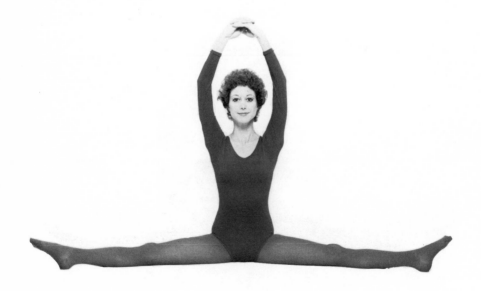

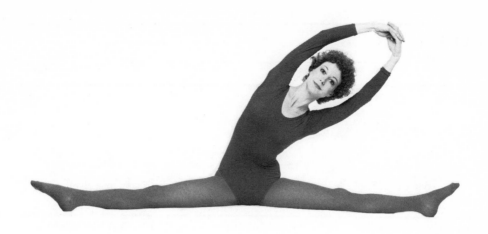

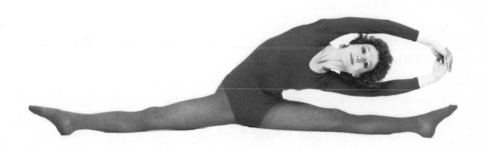

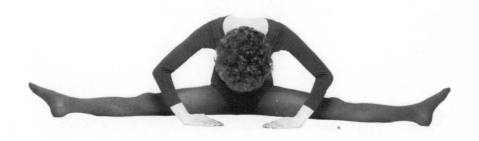

Hips

Ideally speaking, one's hips should be firm, smooth, curved, and well-proportioned. Heaviness in the hips (the area between your waist and buttocks) can truly ruin an otherwise attractive figure. Have you ever found a marvelous pair of trousers that wouldn't slide over your hips comfortably? Or are you constantly letting out the seams of your skirts in order to accommodate your oversized hips? If so, you're among the many who find bathing-suit time depressing and unsettling. Must you camouflage your body in a matronly swim suit instead of indulging in one of the more current and alluring numbers? If the answer is yes, hip-slimming movements are probably a necessity for you.

One must accept the fact, however, that Mother Nature did have something to do with the shape of your hips (as well as the rest of you). It is she who determined whether your pelvis be slim or wide. You'll never be model skinny if you're simply not built long and lean as most models are. If nature has given you a basically shapely, curvaceous form, with hips that might be termed "ample," then you must accept this as your figure type. Wide hips will always be wide just as short legs will always be short, no matter what exercises or beauty rituals you perform. WHAT YOU CAN DO IS WORK ON ACHIEVING YOUR OWN MOST ATTRACTIVE CONTOURS WITHIN THE FRAMEWORK OF YOUR OWN FIGURE TYPE.

Many women with chunky, flabby hips get them purely from bad habits, which means lack of exercise, incorrect diet, and poor posture. Flabbiness in the hips results from improper circulation which is due to lack of exercise. Fatty tissue in the hips can be partially broken up by increased circulation; thus the importance of exercise. Many of my clients who have taken up jogging find their hips and buttocks have shaped up considerably. Again, it is a case of improved circulation and muscle activity.

Many women who formerly have had no figure problems find that, at about age thirty-five, real discipline is necessary in order to keep the lovely shape they had in the past. At approximately this age, overindulgence in food and drink and lack of exercise (or both) really begin to take their toll. That is not to say, however, that younger women don't also suffer from excess weight problems in the hip area.

For women forced into a sedentary life-style (typewriter-trapped or the like), additional emphasis on movement (be it sports, dance, yoga, etc.) is of great importance. Were muscles able to articulate, they would certainly bemoan the debilitating life we force upon them. If you're not experiencing spread in the hips and buttock areas, the exercises in these two sections are ideal as preventive medicine. Should you already be in the process of spreading, these movements can offer a practical, viable means of helping you regain and then maintain more attractive contours.

PLACEMENT: Lie on your back. Extend your legs in front, toes pointed. Rest your hands on your waist.

MOVEMENT: Diagonally lift your right leg to the left. Once it is raised, bounce it further upward four times. Lower the leg and repeat with the left leg.

TOTAL REPETITION: Six times for each leg.

It is important that the shoulders remain stationary during this exercise.

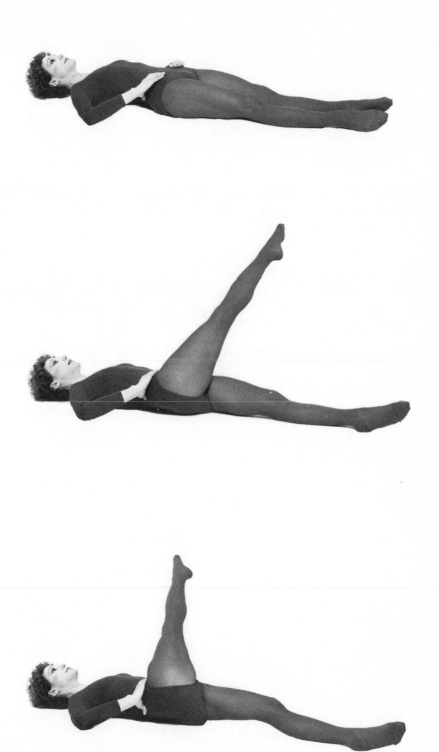

PLACEMENT: Lie on your back with your left leg extended in front. Rest your right foot on your left thigh, knee pointing upward. Place your hands on your waist.

MOVEMENT: Keeping your shoulders stationary and the foot in place, lower the knee as far to the left, then as far to the right as you can. Repeat the total motion six times. Repeat with the left foot on your right leg.

TOTAL REPETITION: Three times for each side.

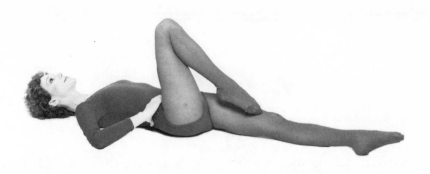

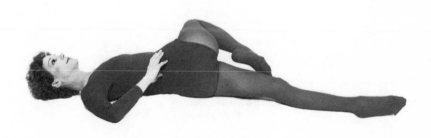

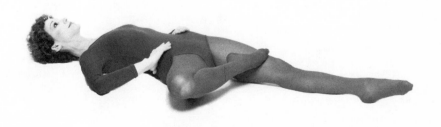

PLACEMENT: Lie on your right side. Use your right elbow and left hand for support. Keep your torso slightly raised.

MOVEMENT: Swing your left leg forward and back, keeping your upper body stationary. On the back swing, contract your buttocks and hold the position for three counts. Repeat eight times. Roll over and repeat on the left side.

TOTAL REPETITION: Three times for each side.

Try to keep the leg swing as level as possible.

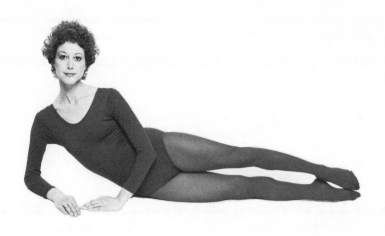

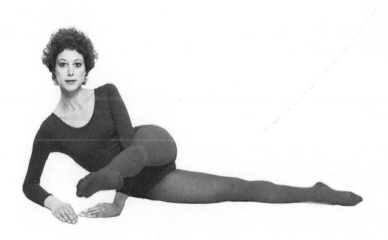

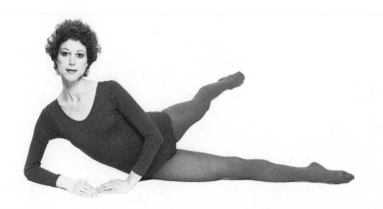

PLACEMENT: Lie on your stomach, legs extended. Place your left hand on top of your right, elbows out. Rest your chin on top of your hands.

MOVEMENT: Keeping your hipbone pressed against the floor, lift your left leg. Swing it to the left four times. Lower the leg and repeat with the right leg, swinging it to the right.

TOTAL REPETITION: Four times for each leg.

Your buttock muscles should be firmly contracted as you swing your leg to the side.

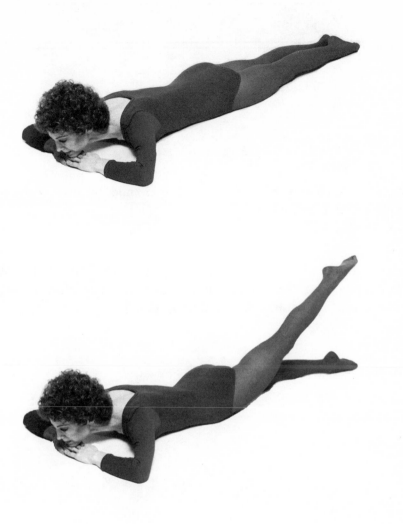

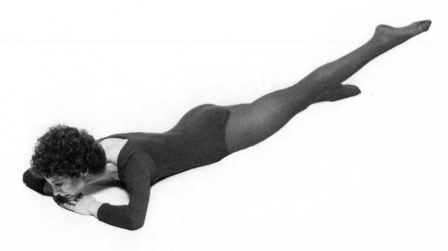

PLACEMENT: Lie on your back with your legs extended in front. Point your toes and place your hands on your hips.

MOVEMENT: Lift your left leg off the floor approximately twelve inches. With the leg in this raised position, swing it all the way to the right, then to the left. Repeat the total swing five times. Repeat with the right leg.

TOTAL REPETITION: Three times for each leg.

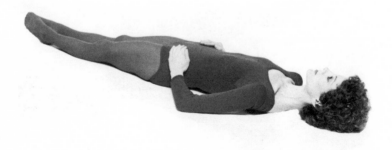

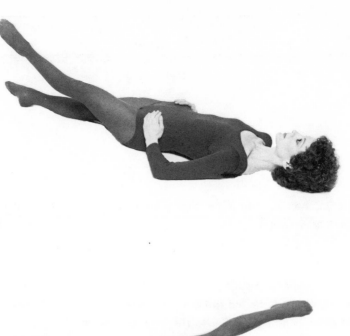

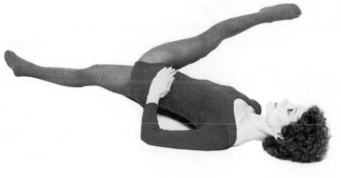

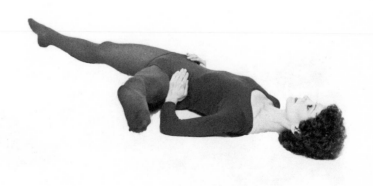

PLACEMENT: Lie on your right side with your right leg extended. Use your right elbow and left hand for support. Bend your left leg so that the knee points forward.

MOVEMENT: Thrust the leg directly back until it is straight. Then swing it to the front before bending it back to the original position. Repeat this semicircular motion, at a fairly rapid tempo, eight times. Roll over and repeat on the left side.

TOTAL REPETITION: Three times for each side.

When thrusting the leg back, contract your buttocks tightly.

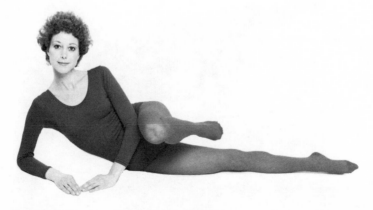

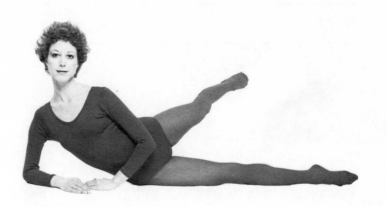

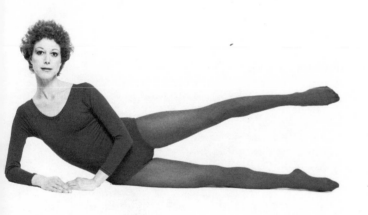

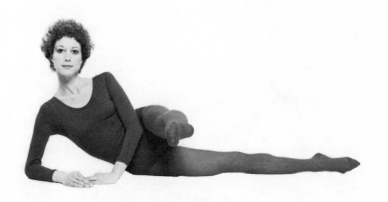

PLACEMENT: Lie on your back with your knees drawn to your chest. Place your hands on your waist.

MOVEMENT: Keeping your shoulders stationary, roll your knees to the left. Extend both legs to the left, on the diagonal. Bend the knees, roll right, and repeat.

TOTAL REPETITION: Eight times for each side.

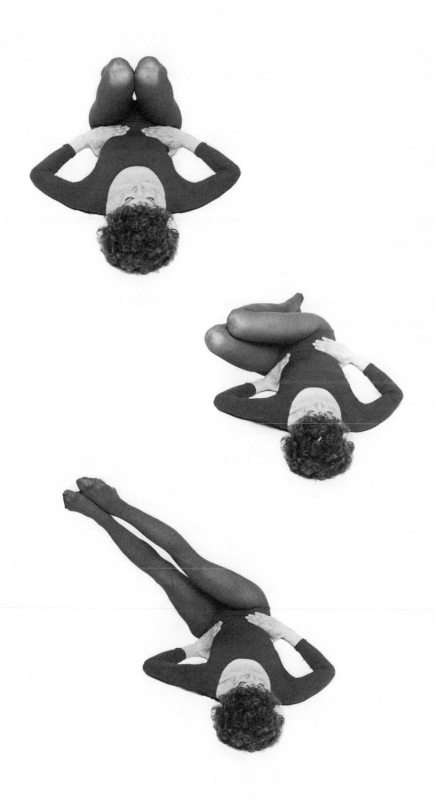

PLACEMENT: Lie on your back with your legs extended in front, toes pointed, heels touching. Place your hands on your waist.

MOVEMENT: Lift the left leg several inches off of the floor and swing it to the left. In this position, force it further back four times. Swing it back into place and repeat with the right leg.

TOTAL REPETITION: Six times for each leg.

It is not necessary to lift the leg too high off the floor. Remember to keep the foot of the leg that is not swinging turned out. This will help to keep your buttocks stationary.

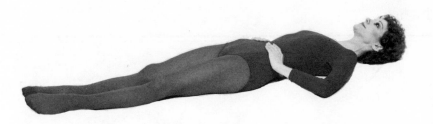

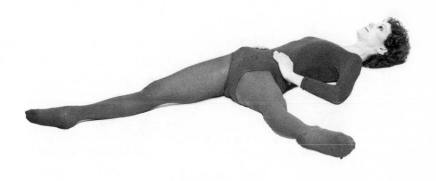

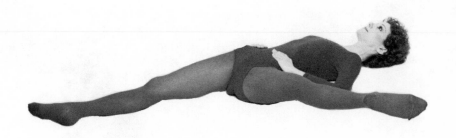

PLACEMENT: Lie on your left side with your left leg extended and your right knee drawn close to your right elbow. Use your left elbow and right hand for support. Turn your upper body to the left.

MOVEMENT: Extend the right leg over the left leg. Lift the right leg, then lower it. Finally bend it back to the original position. The count is: extend—lift —lower—bend. Repeat ten times. Roll over and repeat on the other side.

TOTAL REPETITION: Three times for each side.

This exercise should be done at a fairly rapid tempo.

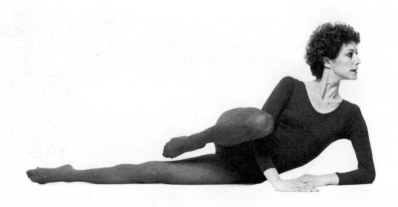

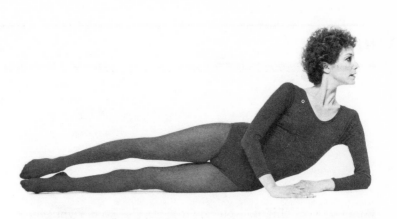

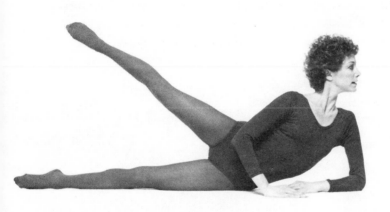

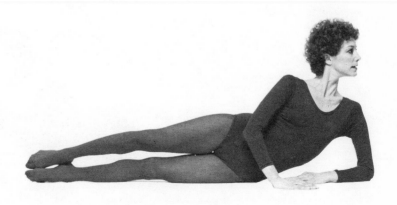

PLACEMENT: Lie on your right side. Use your right elbow and left hand to support your torso which should be slightly raised.

MOVEMENT: Raise your left leg as high as possible. Once it is lifted, raise the right. Hold two counts. Release the right leg, then the left. Repeat six times. Roll over and repeat on the left side.

TOTAL REPETITION: Two times for each side.

Try to raise the second leg as high as the first.

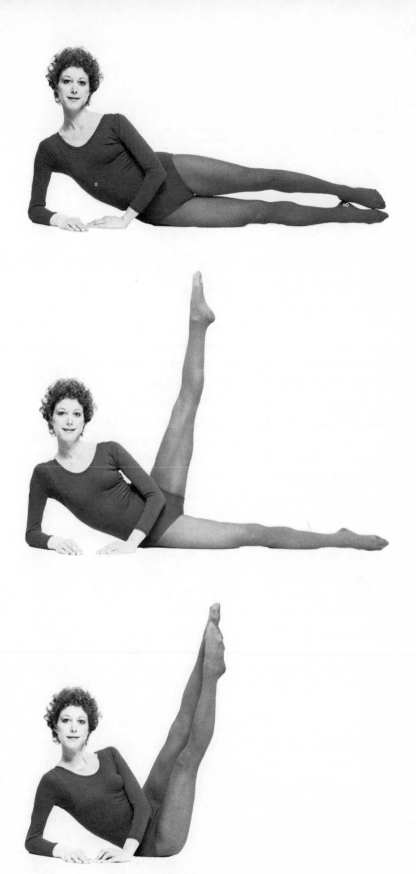

Buttocks

The main danger to the aesthetic appearance of the buttocks is excessive weight. Fat tends to accumulate in certain parts of the body, and in women, in particular, the buttock area is one of the most popular spots for this accumulation. So, too, as one ages, the muscles which extend all over the seat area naturally grow weaker and tend to sag unless special attention is given them. Of course, genetic factors do play a role in the size and shape of your derriere. If your mother and her mom had ample ones, this may be your fate as well.

Aside from practicing the right toners, which work both directly and indirectly on this area, restoring it to its healthiest condition, there are other steps which should be taken as well. Because of the difficulty of bringing this area back to a normal, healthful condition once it has begun to deteriorate, the best advice is to keep off the buttocks as much as possible. Put more movement into your life. Stand more, sit less. Sitting a great deal can only contribute to developing heavy buttocks that are flabby and lacking contour. If you must sit (because of your work), it is important to master the proper way to sit in order to discourage buttock spread. By sitting on your "sitting bones" (instead of on the largest part of your fanny), you can avoid unnecessary enlargement. So, too, it is important when sitting that you avoid crossing your legs (that cuts down vital circulation). In the first place, what exactly are those sitting bones and where are they? They are the bones (called "ischia") underlying the pads of muscle and fat in the buttocks. These are the bones you must learn to sit on. In order to find them, squat like an Indian, resting your buttocks against your heels. In this squatting position, the bones will come in contact with your heels. This is where your weight should be placed when you are sitting.

Sitting too much compresses the tissues in the buttock area thus cutting down on circulation. This causes the buttocks to widen and spread out of proportion. It is most important that you apply yourself sincerely to the buttock and hip toners, as well as to the toners which affect the back of the upper thigh. Contracted voluntarily throughout the day, the buttocks can (with work) become more attractive. Flattened all day (by sitting) and unused, it can only become larger. The function of the toners is to keep the muscles firm and as shapely as the limitations of one's age and natural figure permits.

You must also make yourself a pledge to walk as much as possible instead of driving or riding short distances. Walking can truly have a direct and positive affect on keeping the buttocks firm, lifted, and toned. Pledge not only to walk, but to walk as vigorously as possible, taking long, rhythmic strides. Make walking a part of your daily beauty regimen if at all possible.

Swimming, too, can help trim down a too-large derriere, providing it's done on a regular basis and with the proper energy input. Or you might try simply getting into the pool, holding on to the edge, and kicking your legs in a rapid, scissorlike fashion. Make sure that the entire leg area as well as your buttocks remains under water. Do this flutterlike motion for about thirty seconds, then rest, and repeat several times again. If you don't have access to a pool, you can do flutter kicks right in your bedroom. Lie down on your bed (facing downward) and let just your legs hang over the end of the bed. In this position, start the flutter- or scissor-kick movements. You might do one series in the morning and one in the evening.

Contracting the buttocks is an easy and effective toner. This is done by tightening the buttock muscles as much as possible, holding the contraction for several seconds, then releasing. Repeat this drill for a minute or two, several times a day. You can do it while sitting, standing, or lying down, and no one will even know you're at work on firming your fanny.

PLACEMENT: Lie on your back. Bend your knees and place the soles of your feet on the floor about twelve inches apart and parallel. Rest your arms at your sides.

MOVEMENT: Lift your lower body several inches off of the floor. Contract your buttock muscles tightly. Hold for six counts. Slowly release.

TOTAL REPETITION: Five times.

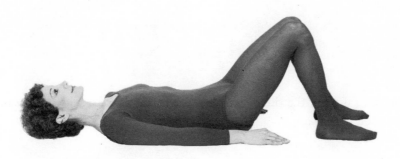

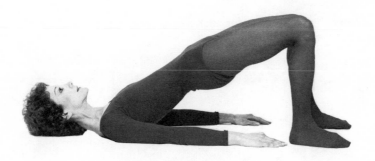

BUTTOCKS 2

PLACEMENT: Lie on the floor with your knees drawn close to your chest. Rest your hands on your waist.

MOVEMENT: Roll your knees to the left, then to the right. Make certain to keep your shoulders stationary.

TOTAL REPETITION: Eight times for each side.

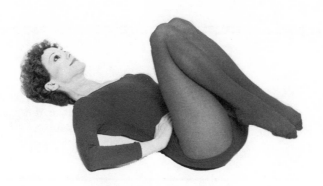

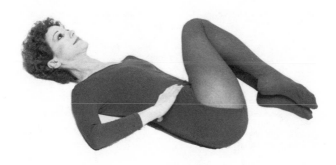

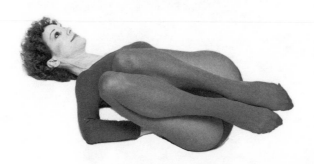

PLACEMENT: Lie on your back. Bend your knees and place the soles of your feet on the floor. Rest your arms at your sides.

MOVEMENT: Bring your right knee toward your chest. Extend the leg upward. Bend it again and extend it forward. Repeat ten times. The count is: bend—extend upward—bend—extend forward. Repeat with the left leg.

TOTAL REPETITION: Two times.

This movement can be done rapidly. When extending the leg forward, keep it close to the floor.

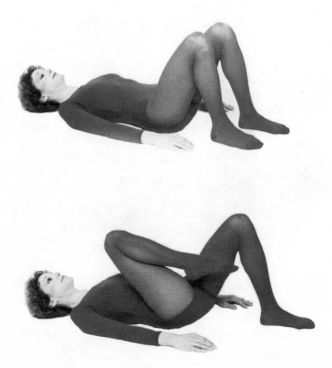

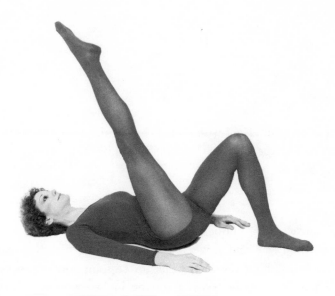

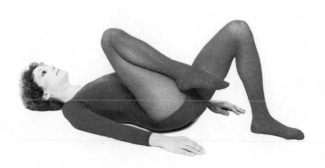

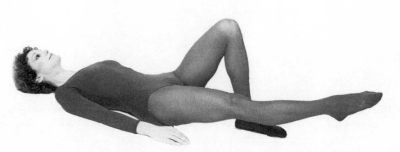

BUTTOCKS 4

PLACEMENT: Lie on your back, with your knees bent, place your feet parallel and about fifteen inches apart. Interlace your fingers behind your head and rest your head in your hands.

MOVEMENT: Contract your buttock muscles and raise your body as high as possible. Use your shoulders and upper back for support. Slowly release until your middle spine is touching the floor. The lower spine and buttocks should remain raised. Then lift your body again to the highest position. Repeat this halfway releasing motion four times. Release all the way to the floor and draw your knees to your chest. Rock your knees forward and back four times, keeping your head on the floor.

TOTAL REPETITION: Two times.

As you uncurl from the lifted position, keep contracting your abdominals.

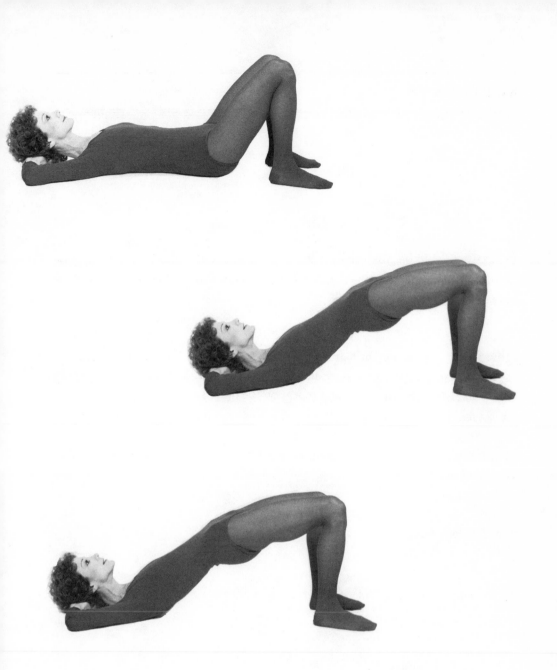

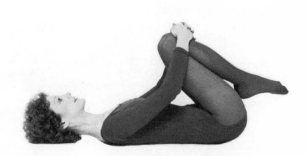

PLACEMENT: Lie on your right side. Leaning on your right elbow, keep your torso slightly raised. Use your left hand for support. Extend your left leg behind the right, toes resting on the floor.

MOVEMENT: Keeping the left foot pointed downward, lift and lower the leg five times. Next turn your upper body toward your right shoulder and repeat the leg lift five times. Roll over and repeat on the other side.

TOTAL REPETITION: Two times for each side.

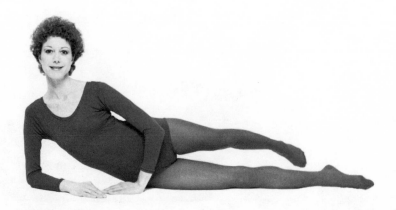

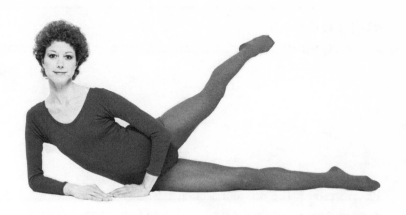

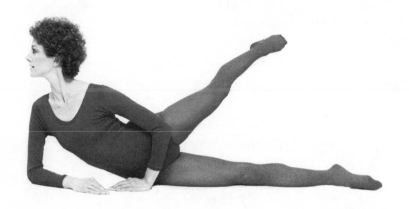

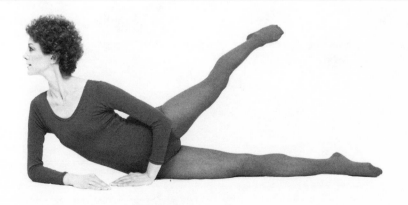

PLACEMENT: Lie on your stomach with your legs extended. Rest your right hand on top of your left and your chin on top of your hands.

MOVEMENT: Lift your right leg, toes pointed. Keeping the leg raised, bend and straighten it six times. Lower the leg and repeat on the left.

TOTAL REPETITION: Three times for each leg.

Try to keep your hipbone pressed against the floor while the leg is lifted.

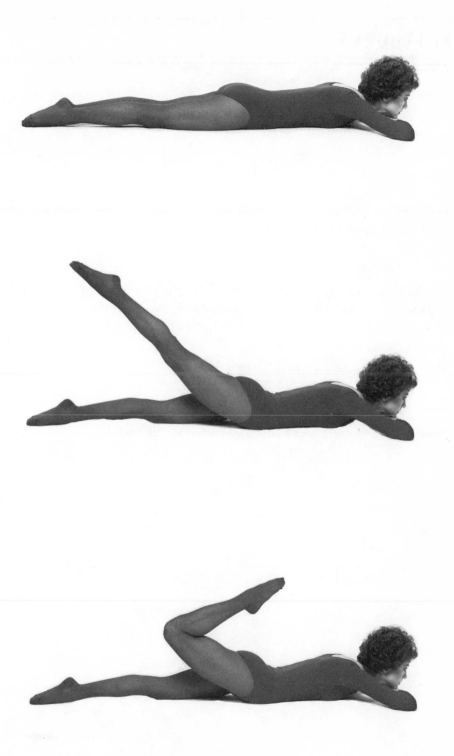

PLACEMENT: Lie on your stomach with your legs extended. Rest your right hand on top of your left and your chin on top of your hands.

MOVEMENT: Keeping your hipbone down, lift the right leg, then the left. Hold for two counts. Release both legs simultaneously.

TOTAL REPETITION: Eight times.

Remember to contract your buttock muscles as you lift your legs.

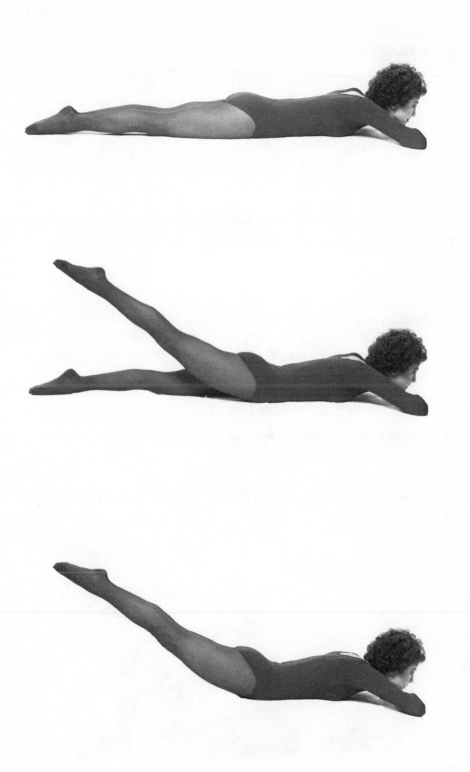

PLACEMENT: Lie on your back, with your knees bent. Place the soles of your feet on the floor about ten inches apart and parallel. Rest your arms at your sides.

MOVEMENT: Contract your buttocks and lift your body as high as possible. In this raised position, slide your right foot forward until the leg is straight. The right hip should tilt downward. Slide the leg back and repeat on the left leg. Center yourself and slowly release to the floor.

TOTAL REPETITION: Eight times.

On the releasing motion, make certain your buttocks touch the floor last.

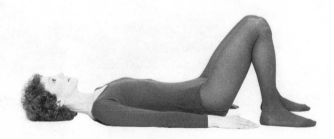

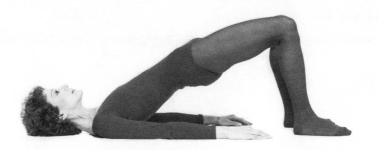

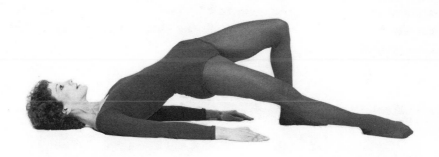

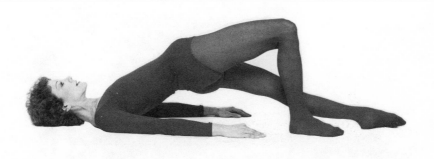

PLACEMENT: Lie on your stomach with your legs extended. Place your left hand on top of your right.

MOVEMENT: Lift both legs as high as possible. In this raised position, scissor-kick them eight times. Lower both legs simultaneously.

TOTAL REPETITION: Three times.

This motion is similar to a flutter kick.

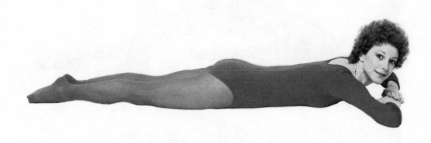

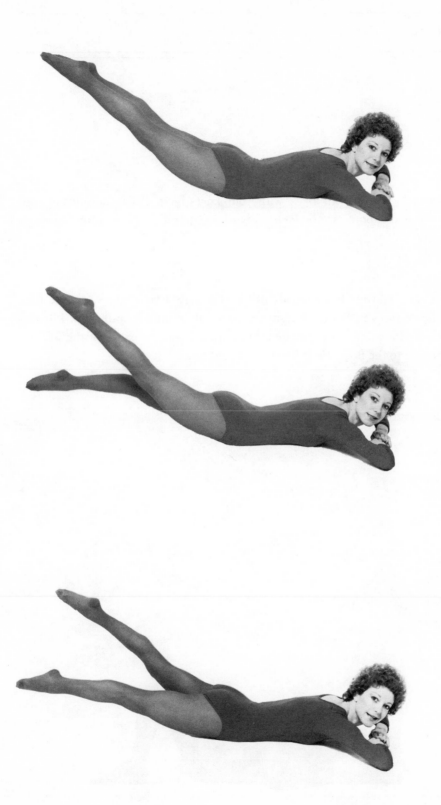

PLACEMENT: Lie on your back with your knees bent. Place the soles of your feet on the floor about twelve inches apart and parallel. Place your hands on your waist.

MOVEMENT: Slowly lift your body off the floor. Rest your elbows on the floor for additional support. Slide the right leg on the floor until it is straight. Lift and lower the leg four times, toes pointed. Slide it back and repeat with the left leg. Slowly release to the floor. Your buttocks should touch last.

TOTAL REPETITION: Three times for each leg.

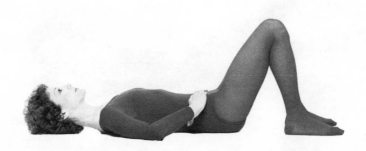

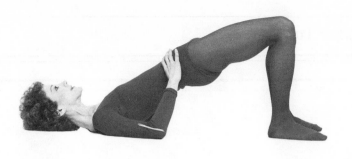

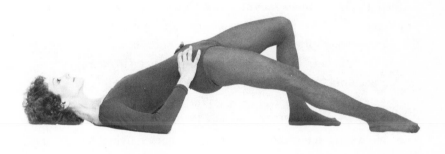

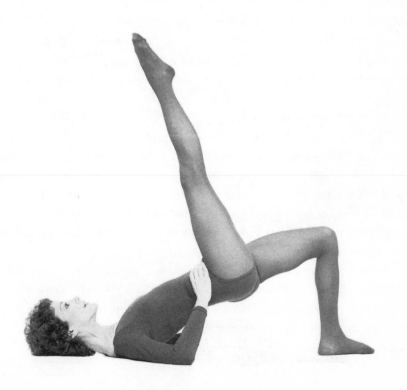

Thighs

Since the thighs are four dimensional, problems in this area can be single or multiple. The outer thigh tends to bulge, the inner thigh to sag, and the front and back to become rippled and flabby. The thighs seem to be the number one trouble spot. At about age thirty-five, many women begin to notice deterioration of their thighs, both in condition· and in appearance. For many, this deterioration seems to take place at an all-too-rapid rate. Similar to the upper arms, the thighs (especially the inner and outer portions) are prone to flab. The correction for this flabby condition depends on diet (to reduce fat and prevent its further accumulation) plus a regimen of the correct thigh toners.

Weight in the thigh area is, unfortunately, difficult to reduce. It may be that you've dieted faithfully and lost in other areas (bosom, face, midriff) but your thighs have remained oversized and unattractive. The one and only answer for improving the over-all appearance of your thighs is regular exercise. Walk, jog, swim, jump rope, or bicycle. Or, perhaps, take up a movement course in something you've never tried before—tap, ballet, or maybe fencing. Add to this the correct thigh toners and you'll be able to redistribute the flesh somewhat, attaining more attractive contours. It is through the proper balance of contracting and stretching movements that more slender thighs can be developed. Dance and yoga classes can be extremely beneficial for streamlining the thighs, no matter what shape they were born to.

The thighs also respond well to water exercises. Pushing against the weight of the water gives additional effectiveness to leg movements. And because the rest of your body is buoyed up, exercising in water reduces over-all body strain. One of my favorite thigh exercises can actually be done right in the bathtub. Sit and face the outer rim of the tub. Place the soles of your feet together. Rest your hands on the tub rim. Slowly push your knees down as far as they will go. Hold this position for five seconds, then release, allowing your knees to lift. I particularly enjoy stretching and toning in the tub because the water of a bath (especially when I soak in an aromatic herbal mix) can be so very restorative. Besides, why not maximize tub time while you minimize your figure flaws? One note of caution however: do treat yourself to a good rubber mat for the bottom of the tub in order to assure safety while tub toning.

A thigh toner I often do while sitting on the edge of the pool is both easy and very effective. Let your legs dangle so that the lower parts, up to the knees, are under water. Straighten the right leg, then slowly lift it out of the water, toes pointed. Lift it as high as possible, then bounce it upward four times. Lower the leg and repeat on the left side. Repeat ten times. You may find that you will tire at first, but as your muscles get firm, you'll be able to increase the repetitions considerably.

Spending too much time sitting on your derriere is detrimental to the thighs as well as to the hips and buttocks. Sitting causes compression of the thigh tissues and thus restricts vital circulation. That is why women with sedentary jobs are so often prone to oversized thighs, hips, and buttocks. If your job keeps you in a chair for extended periods of time, make an effort at various times during the day to simply get up and stretch. Just shake out your legs vigorously in order to set your circulation in motion. Even a minute or two of movement can make a difference. While at your desk, refrain from crossing your legs. It's just another means of cutting down on the blood flow and inviting unwanted flab.

The sedentary woman must also make an effort to incorporate other movement into her day, since her muscles simply do not receive sufficient use during the work week. Perhaps a morning swim or jog before work. If that's not possible, a lunchtime dance or yoga class might be the answer for revving up circulation. When none of these alternatives are possible, a brisk walk for ten or fifteen minutes can be beneficial.

One pleasurable way to activate your blood flow and rev up vital circulation in your thighs is to spend ten or fifteen minutes on a slant board. If you don't own an actual slant board, your ironing board will do just fine. Simply prop up the narrow end of the board so that it is approximately fifteen inches off of the floor. Make certain that the board is propped up on something stable. Then lie on top with your feet elevated and resting on the narrow end of the board. Close your eyes and relax. I generally place a small pillow under my head and occasionally a skin mask on my face. It's a wonderful time to take advantage of an at-home facial. Relaxing on a slant board can be particularly soothing for a woman who's on her feet for hours at a time. Many of my clients have discovered that a mere ten minutes on the board can do wonders for preparing them for a busy night on the town.

As you flip through the pages of this book, you will notice many exercises performed in a sitting position with the legs extended to the sides. This is called a "second-position stretch" and is extremely beneficial for inner-thigh toning. Should flabby inner thighs be your personal figure flaw, you might wish to concentrate on those second-position movements even if they appear in other sections of the book.

The condition commonly known as "saddlebags" describes the accumulation of fat on the outer thigh. Again, the correct toners can help to remedy this condition when practiced faithfully. Leg swings such as the ones that appear on pages 89 and 131 are extremely beneficial. For toning and tightening the front of the thigh, leg lifting and kicking movements work well. It might be comforting and encouraging to know that while you firm your thighs with the exercises in this chapter, you will at the same time be exercising your knees, ankles, and even your feet. This means you can develop strength and flexibility in your entire leg as you streamline and slenderize your thighs. Remember, a woman's thighs do not spread and weaken with age because they're "supposed to" but instead because they're simply neglected.

THIGHS 1

PLACEMENT: Lie on your back. Extend your right leg in front and rest your left foot on the floor. Place your hands on your waist.

MOVEMENT: Bounce the right leg up and down three times, raising it only halfway and touching it to the floor each time. On the fourth count, lift the leg as high as possible. The count is: bounce—bounce—bounce—lift. Repeat five times. Repeat on the left leg.

TOTAL REPETITION: Three times for each leg.

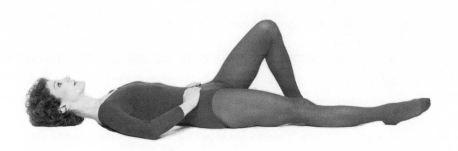

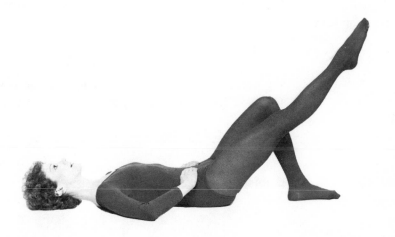

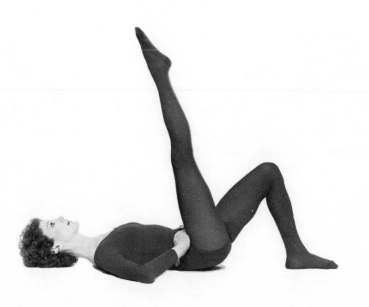

THIGHS 2

PLACEMENT: Lie on your back. Extend your right leg in front. Bend your left knee, place your left foot on the floor, and tilt your left knee slightly to the left. Rest your hands on your waist.

MOVEMENT: Lift the right leg diagonally to the left, toes pointed. Repeat six times. Next, flex your right foot and lift it directly upward six times. Repeat with the left leg.

TOTAL REPETITION: Three times for each leg.

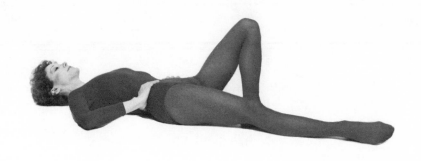

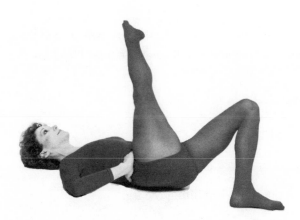

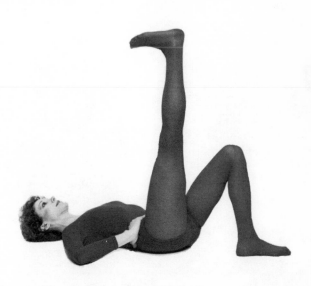

PLACEMENT: Sit with your legs extended in front. Lift your arms upward, palms facing in.

MOVEMENT: Lift the right leg five times, then lift the left five times. Next, release your body forward from the hips and reach for your toes. Hold for five counts.

TOTAL REPETITION: Three times.

Try to keep your back as erect as possible when lifting the leg.

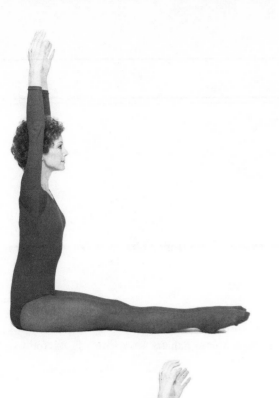

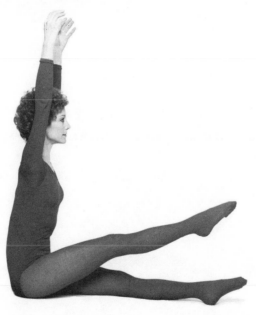

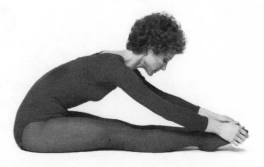

PLACEMENT: Sit with your legs extended in front. Place your hands on your waist.

MOVEMENT: Lift the right leg several inches off the floor. Swing the leg to the right, then swing it left, crossing over the left leg. Repeat four times. Lower the leg and repeat with the left leg.

TOTAL REPETITION: Three times for each leg.

Try to keep your body as stationary as possible when swinging the leg.

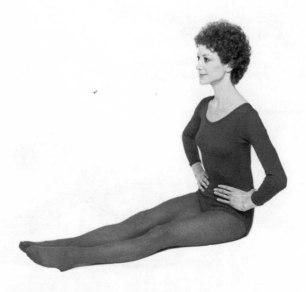

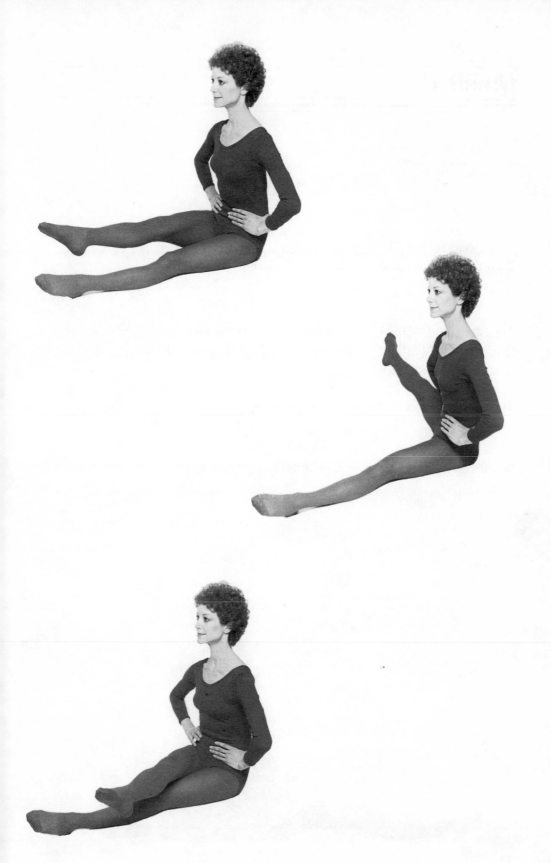

PLACEMENT: Lie flat on your back with your left leg extended on the floor. Bend the right knee and clasp your hands around the right calf.

MOVEMENT: Keeping your hands in place, straighten and bend the leg eight times. Repeat with the left leg.

TOTAL REPETITION: Three times for each leg.

In order to make this exercise more difficult, try clasping your hands nearer your ankle.

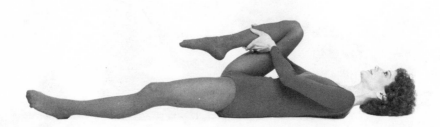

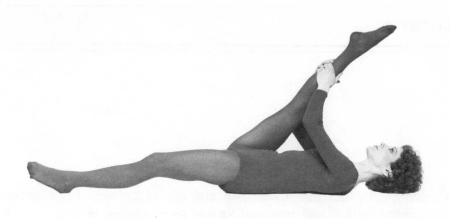

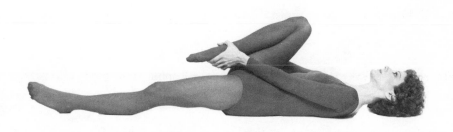

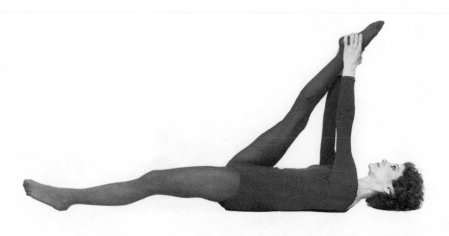

PLACEMENT: Sit with your knees apart and the soles of your feet together. Clasp your left hand around your toes. Extend your right arm in front at chest level, palm down.

MOVEMENT: Reach forward four times, pressing your knees down. Repeat, holding your toes with your right hand and extending your left arm. Next place both hands on your feet. Round your back and bounce the knees up and down four times.

TOTAL REPETITION: Three times.

Be certain to keep your buttocks stationary as you reach forward.

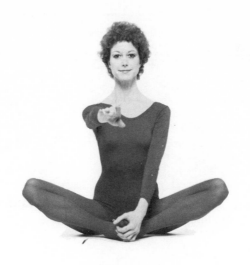

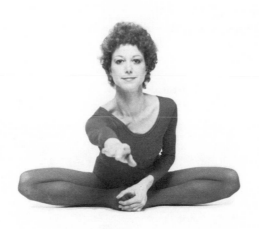

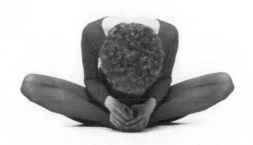

PLACEMENT: Lie on your back. Extend your legs upward so that they form a V. Rest your arms on the floor, palms down.

MOVEMENT: Slowly lower your legs to the sides until they are as far apart as possible. Hold this position for four slow counts. Then resume the original position. Repeat five times. Next, hug your knees to your chest and hold five counts.

TOTAL REPETITION: Three times.

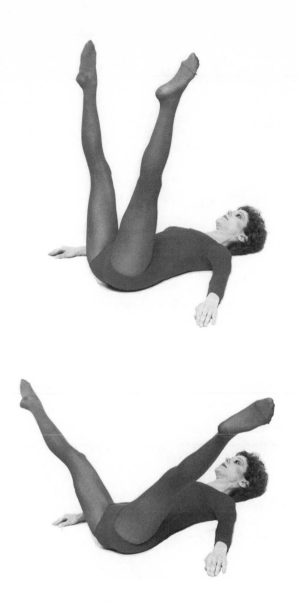

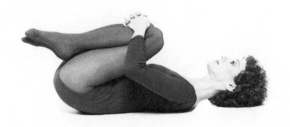

PLACEMENT: Sit erect with your legs extended to the sides, toes pointed. Place your palms on the floor between your legs.

MOVEMENT: Slide your hands forward as you simultaneously lower your upper body. Hold for three counts. Straighten to the starting position.

TOTAL REPETITION: Eight times.

This movement can also be done with the feet flexed. Try it both ways.

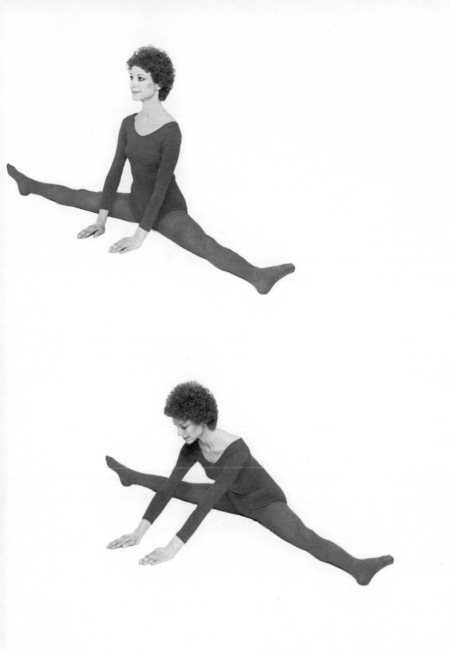

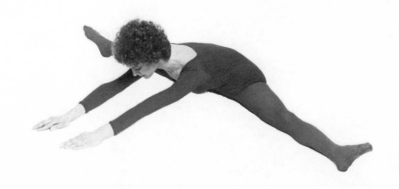

PLACEMENT: Sit with your left foot close to your body. Bend your right leg. Clasp your right hand around your right heel.

MOVEMENT: Extend the right leg in front until it is straight and extended as high as possible. Bend the leg, then extend it to the right side. Repeat this sequence five times. Repeat with the left leg.

TOTAL REPETITION: Three times for each leg.

Try to keep your back as erect as possible while doing this exercise.

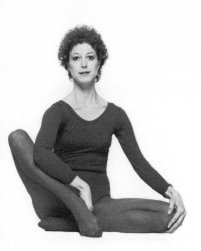

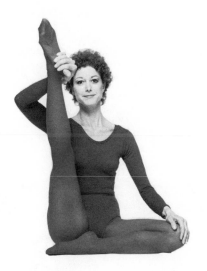

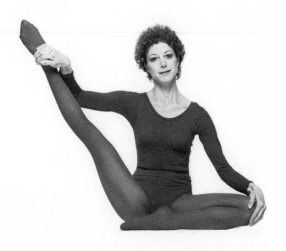

PLACEMENT: Lie on your left side, legs straight. Support yourself with your left elbow and right hand. Keep your torso slightly lifted. Extend your right leg behind and as high as possible.

MOVEMENT: Keeping the leg in a raised position, bend and straighten it ten times. Roll over and repeat on the right side with the left leg.

TOTAL REPETITION: Three times for each side.

This movement can be done fairly rapidly. Keep the toes pointed and your buttocks firmly contracted.

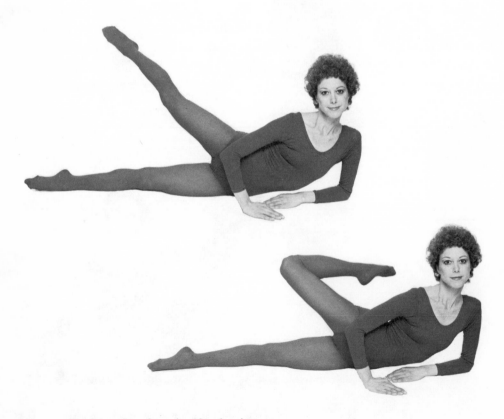

_3_

Regimens

All the exercises in these regimens have been taken from Chapter 2 or are slight variations of those movements. Each regimen includes four exercises (two per body area) and has been carefully chosen in order to assist you in working on the most common combined figure faults. These effective routines can be practiced in addition to the toners in Chapter 2 _once you have perfected the toners you are in need of_. Each regimen should take approximately five minutes to complete. You can thus create your own sequences (five, ten, fifteen, etc. minutes) by stringing several regimens together. Practice the exercises as indicated in the illustrations, according to the repetitions required. After two weeks' time, you may, if you wish, begin to increase the repetitions gradually until the numbers have eventually doubled. In this way, these regimens can serve as a beneficial maintenance program.

Abdominals/Hips

Flabby abdominals coupled with oversized hips comprise a common combined figure condition for many women. During pregnancy, this condition often becomes more critical. Poor postural habits due to weight gain cause the abdominals to become lax and flaccid. As for the hips, they tend to become thick and heavy as a result of inactivity and improper body alignment. So, too, during pregnancy, the hips seem to act as food magnets, broadcasting each and every eating splurge.

ABDOMINALS 1

PLACEMENT: Lie on your back, knees bent close to your chest. Rest your arms at your sides, palms down.

MOVEMENT: Keeping the left knee in place, extend your right leg until it is straight and several inches off of the floor. Hold for three counts. Bring the leg back into position and repeat with the left leg. Repeat eight times. Draw your knees to your chest and rock them forward and back four times.

TOTAL REPETITION: Two times. ·

As you extend the leg forward, make certain that your abdominals are contracted.

ABDOMINALS 2

PLACEMENT: Lie on the floor with your right leg extended in front. Rest your left foot on the floor. Extend your arms on the floor over your head.

MOVEMENT: Lift your head, neck, and shoulders off the floor. Simultaneously swing your arms forward. Hold for two counts, then slowly release. Repeat four times with your right leg extended, then four times with the left.

TOTAL REPETITION: Three times.

Try to maintain the contraction at the maximum stress point. Do not sit up all the way. Stop when your middle back is no longer resting on the floor.

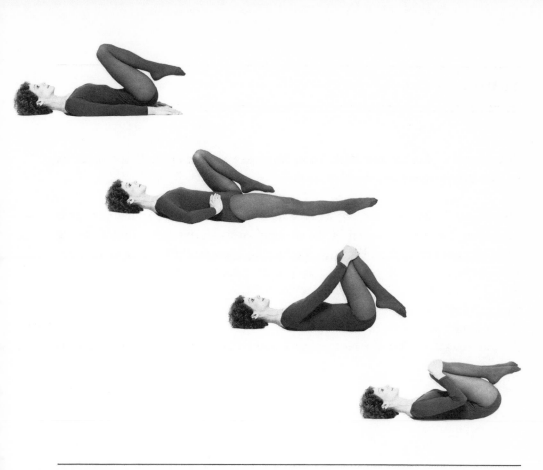

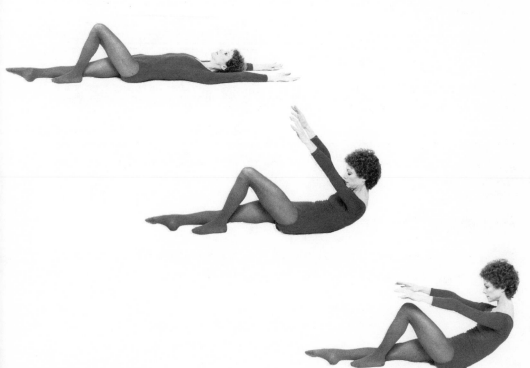

HIPS 1

PLACEMENT: Lie on your right side. Use your right elbow and left hand for support. Keep your torso slightly raised.

MOVEMENT: Swing your left leg forward and back, keeping your upper body stationary. On the back swing, contract your buttocks and hold the position for three counts. Repeat eight times. Roll over and repeat on the left side.

TOTAL REPETITION: Three times for each side.

Try to keep the leg swing as level as possible.

HIPS 2

PLACEMENT: Lie on your back with your knees drawn to your chest. Place your hands on your waist.

MOVEMENT: Keeping your shoulders stationary, roll your knees to the left. Extend both legs to the left, on the diagonal. Bend the knees, roll right, and repeat.

TOTAL REPETITION: Eight times for each side.

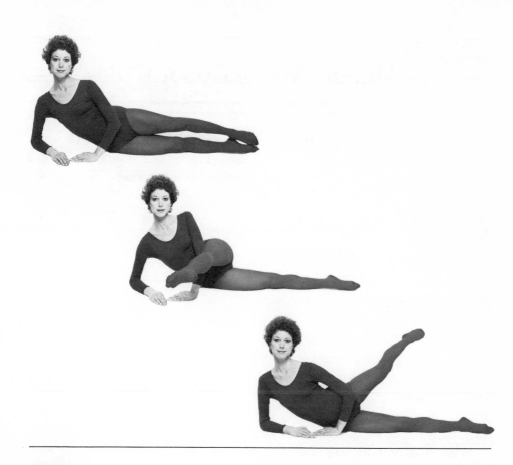

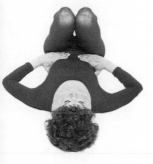

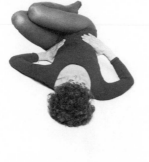

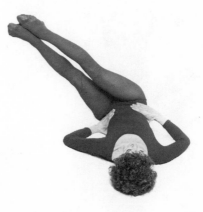

Thighs/Upper Arms/Bosom

Flabby thighs and sagging upper arms and bosom are often caused by the combination of neglect (lack of movement) and excess weight. The sagging skin is a result of the gradual loss of muscles and is frequently most evident in the upper arms and thighs (especially the inner portion). Exercising both areas is imperative in order to prevent the loss of active cells and thus the accumulation of fat. Remember, where you sag first is partly determined by what you do (or don't do) with your body. USE IT OR LOSE IT! It's as simple as that.

THIGHS 1

PLACEMENT: Sit with your knees apart and the soles of your feet together. Clasp your left hand around your toes. Extend your right arm in front at chest level, palm down.

MOVEMENT: Reach forward with your right arm four times, pressing your knees down. Repeat, holding your toes with your right hand and extending your left arm. Next, place both hands on your feet. Round your back and bounce the knees up and down four times.

TOTAL REPETITION: Three times.

Be certain to keep your buttocks stationary as you reach forward.

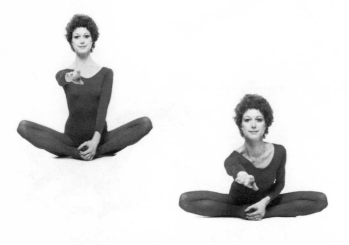

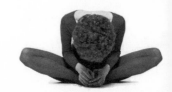

THIGHS 2

PLACEMENT: Sit erect with your legs extended to the sides, toes pointed. Place your palms on the floor between your legs.

MOVEMENT: Slide your hands forward as you simultaneously lower your upper body. Hold for three counts. Straighten to the starting position.

TOTAL REPETITION: Eight times.

This movement can also be done with the feet flexed. Try it both ways.

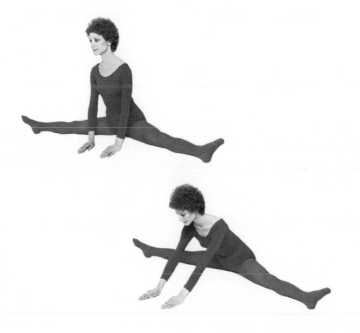

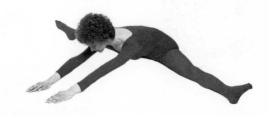

UPPER ARMS/BOSOM 1

PLACEMENT: Sit with your knees apart and the soles of your feet together. Rest your hands on your toes.

MOVEMENT: Stretch upward with your right arm. Reach forward, stretching as far as possible. Next lift your arm and body until your back is straight. Lower the arm and repeat with the left arm.

TOTAL REPETITION: Six times for each arm.

As you reach forward, press your knees down and keep your buttocks stationary.

UPPER ARMS/BOSOM 2

PLACEMENT: Sit erect with your legs extended to the sides. Clasp your hands behind your body, fingers interlaced.

MOVEMENT: Round your back and lower your head as close to the floor as possible. At the same time, lift your arms. Hold for three counts. Lift your body back to position as you lower your arms.

TOTAL REPETITION: Ten times.

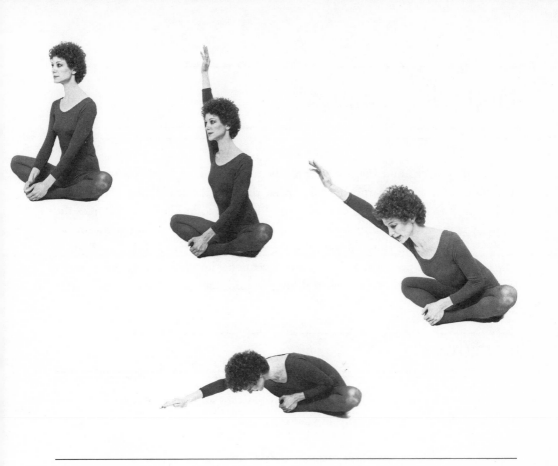

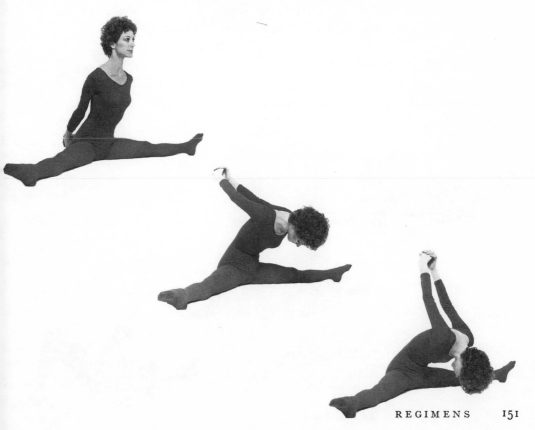

Buttocks/Thighs

Oversized buttocks and thighs can truly be a problem, especially when fashion dictates close-fitting apparel. If you've been through the frustration of trying to find trousers that fit properly or a skirt that doesn't require letting out across the fanny, you're probably somewhat "bottom-heavy." Sitting too much or incorrectly can be a main cause of spread since it cuts down on circulation. Regular physical activity, performed at a fairly strenuous level, will help slim heavy thighs and reduce excess buttock padding, in addition to improving your overall well-being.

BUTTOCKS 1

PLACEMENT: Lie on your back. Bend your knees and place the soles of your feet on the floor. Rest your arms at your sides.

MOVEMENT: Bring your right knee toward your chest. Extend the leg upward. Bend it again and extend it forward. Repeat ten times. The count is: bend—extend upward—bend—extend forward. Repeat with the left leg.

TOTAL REPETITION: Two times.

This movement can be done rapidly. When extending the leg forward, keep it close to the floor.

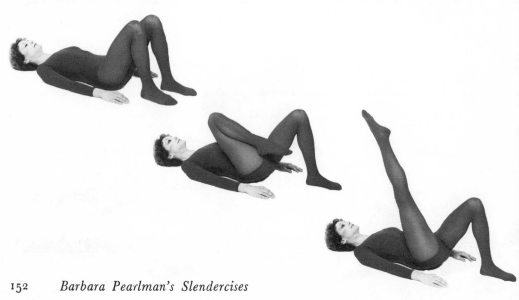

BUTTOCKS 2

PLACEMENT: Lie on your right side. Lean on your right elbow. Keep your torso slightly raised. Use your left hand for support. Extend your left leg behind the right, toes resting on the floor.

MOVEMENT: Keeping the left foot pointed downward, lift and lower the leg five times. Next turn your upper body toward your right shoulder and repeat the left leg lift five times. Roll over and repeat on the other side.

TOTAL REPETITION: Two times for each side.

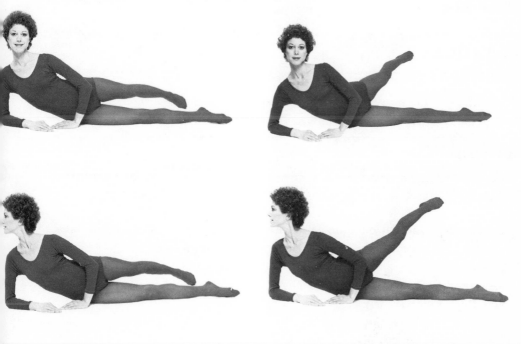

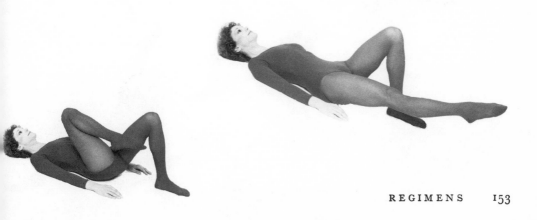

THIGHS 1

PLACEMENT: Lie on your back. Extend your right leg in front, bend your left knee. Place your left foot on the floor and tilt your left knee slightly to the left. Rest your hands on your waist.

MOVEMENT: Lift the right leg diagonally to the left, toes pointed. Repeat six times. Next flex your right foot and lift it directly upward six times. Repeat with the left leg.

TOTAL REPETITION: Three times for each leg.

THIGHS 2

PLACEMENT: Lie flat on your back with your left leg extended on the floor. Bend the right knee and clasp your hands around the right calf.

MOVEMENT: Keeping your hands in place, straighten and bend the leg eight times. Repeat with the left leg.

TOTAL REPETITION: Three times for each leg.

In order to make this exercise more difficult, try clasping your hands nearer to your ankle.

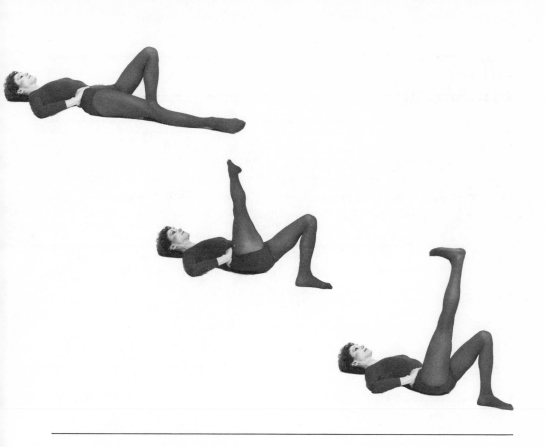

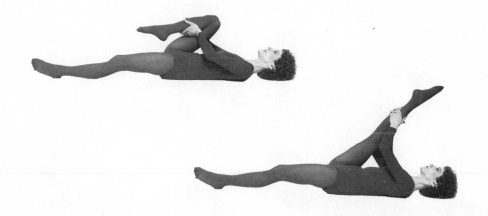

Hips/Buttocks

Despite years of neglect, plus a conviction you may have that your problem is hopeless, you can alter the shape of your hips and buttocks. In the majority of cases, it seems that heavy hips are in frequent partnership with a spreading derriere. Generally, most exercises that are designed to firm the buttocks will also recontour the hips. You can, if you're disciplined and patient, redistribute the flesh and trim away excess flab. The best way? Activity! Move, move, move. Try to sit less. Make every effort to rev up your circulation. It's the only way to reduce heaviness in the hip and buttock areas.

HIPS 1

PLACEMENT: Lie on your stomach, legs extended. Place your right hand on top of your left, elbows out. Rest your chin on top of your hands.

MOVEMENT: Keeping your hipbone pressed against the floor, lift your left leg. Swing it to the left four times. Lower the leg and repeat with the right leg, swinging it to the right.

TOTAL REPETITION: Four times for each leg.

Your buttock muscles should be firmly contracted as you swing your leg to the side.

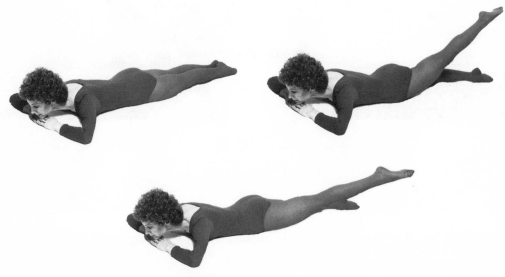

HIPS 2

PLACEMENT: Lie on your right side with your right leg extended. Use your right elbow and left hand for support. Bend your left leg so that the knee points forward.

MOVEMENT: Thrust the leg directly back until it is straight. Then swing it to the front before bending it back to the original position. Repeat this semicircular motion, at a fairly rapid tempo, eight times. Roll over and repeat on the left side.

TOTAL REPETITION: Three times for each side.

When thrusting the leg back, contract your buttocks tightly.

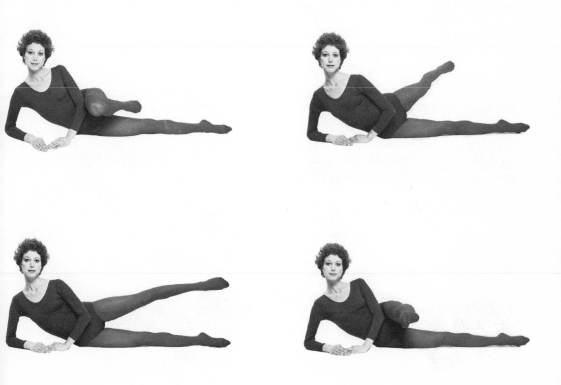

BUTTOCKS 1

PLACEMENT: Lie on the floor with your knees drawn close to your chest. Rest your hands on your waist.

MOVEMENT: Roll your knees to the left, then to the right. Make certain to keep your shoulders stationary.

TOTAL REPETITION: Eight times for each side.

BUTTOCKS 2

PLACEMENT: Lie on your stomach, legs extended. Rest your right hand on top of your left and your chin on top of your hands.

MOVEMENT: Keeping your hipbone down, lift the right leg, then the left. Hold for two counts. Release both legs simultaneously.

TOTAL REPETITION: Eight times.

Remember to contract your buttock muscles as you lift your legs.

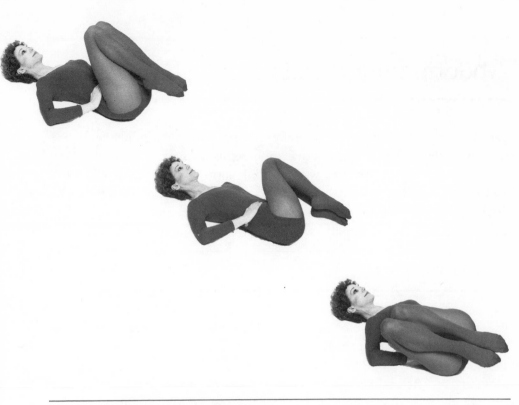

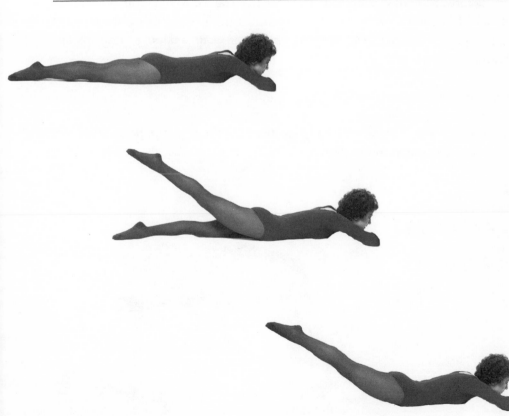

Abdominals/Waist

Lack of exercise and movement generally results in flabby abdominals and a less-than-streamlined waist. Excess weight also seems to have a way of settling around the midsection. The best way to whittle away at your waistline and tone your abdominals is to move more and exercise with twisting, turning, stretching, reaching motions. Posture, too, plays an important role. Hold your torso high and immediately your abdominals and waist will appear more attractive.

ABDOMINALS 1

PLACEMENT: Sit with your knees bent. Place the soles of your feet parallel and about twelve inches apart. Extend your arms in front at chest level.

MOVEMENT: Release your body halfway back. At the same time, slide your left leg forward until it is straight. Hold for two counts. Resume the original position and repeat with your right leg. Repeat ten times. Then extend both legs in front, round your back, and rest your hands on your ankles. Bounce up and down four times.

TOTAL REPETITION: Two times.

Remember not to release your body too far back. Stop at the point when you are supported by your lower spine.

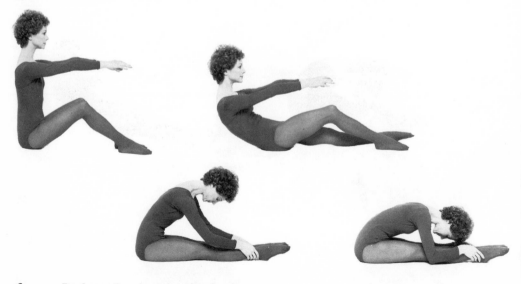

ABDOMINALS 2

PLACEMENT: Lie on your back, legs extended in front. Rest your arms on the floor over your head.

MOVEMENT: Roll up to a halfway sit-up position with your knees bent, toes pointed and resting on the floor. Your back should be rounded. As you lift your body, your arms will naturally swing forward. Next, slide your legs on the floor and simultaneously reach for your ankles. Finally, uncurl slowly back to the floor. The count is: lift—stretch—uncurl.

TOTAL REPETITION: Ten times.

Try to keep this movement fluid and controlled. As you release back to the floor, contract your abdominal and buttock muscles.

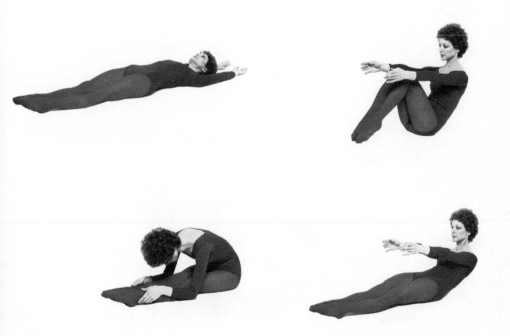

WAIST 1

PLACEMENT: Sit with your legs extended as far to the sides as possible. Twist your upper body to the right. Extend your arms in front of your body at chest level.

MOVEMENT: Stretch forward from your waist. Then pull all the way back. Repeat this forward and back motion four times. Twist to the left and repeat.

TOTAL REPETITION: Three times for each side.

It is important that you keep your buttocks stationary on the forward-stretching motion.

WAIST 2

PLACEMENT: Sit with your legs extended to the sides, knees bent. Rest your hands on your legs and the soles of your feet on the floor.

MOVEMENT: Lean to the right. Slide your right hand toward your right foot as your left arm arches overhead, palm up. Bounce up and down three times. Return to center and repeat, leaning to the left.

TOTAL REPETITION: Six times for each side.

This movement can also be done as a single stretch, without the bounce. After completion of this exercise, bring your legs together and gently bounce them up and down several times.

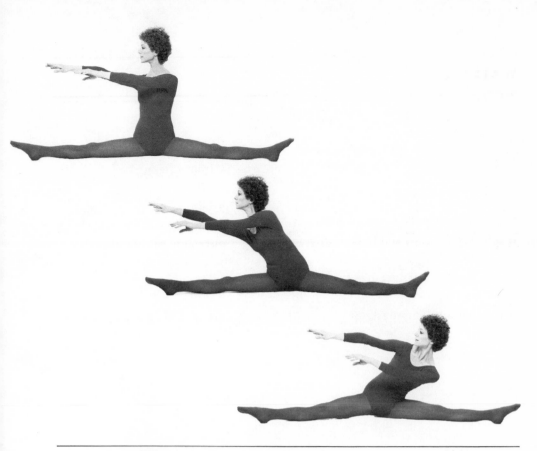

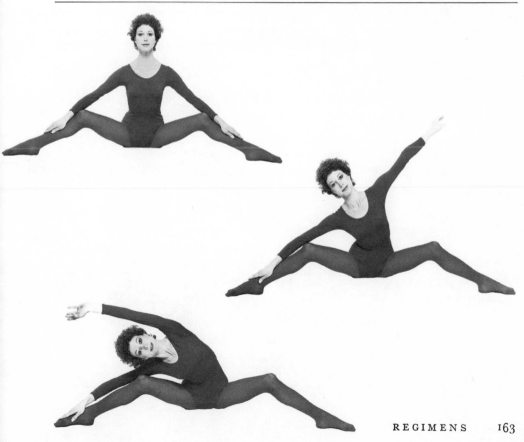

4

Barbara's Body
Bonus

Done on a fairly regular basis, this seven-minute Body Bonus routine can help you become more slimber. The Body Bonus consists of ten exercises that follow a definite and important sequential pattern. Thus muscles are used in a particular way, in a particular manner. This mini-program is composed of five primary positions. For each position, there are two movements. The ten exercises should be taken in sequence and, if at all possible, for the number of repetitions indicated. The Body Bonus is multipurposed. It can be used in addition to the toners and regimens. Or it can be used in other ways—as a quick Morning Awakener, as an Anytime Energy Booster, or simply as an effective preparation for the rigors of more strenuous activity.

PLACEMENT: Stand with your feet wide apart and slightly turned out. Extend your arms overhead.

MOVEMENT: Stretch upward, first with your right arm, then with your left. Repeat eight times. Next, round your back and swing your arms back and forth between your legs three times. On the fourth count, swing your arms forward and assume your original position.

TOTAL REPETITION: Three times.

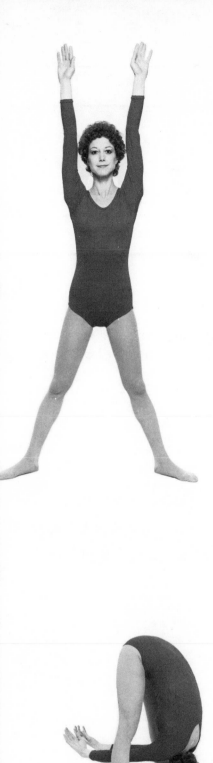

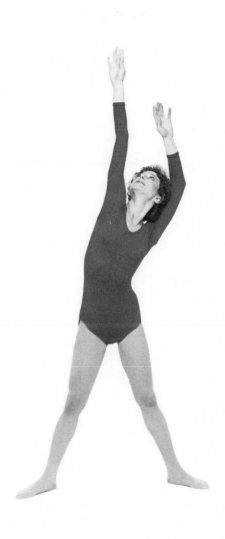

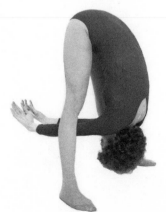

PLACEMENT: Stand with your feet wide apart and turned out. Place your hands on your hips.

MOVEMENT: Lunge to the right. Simultaneously lift your arms overhead, crossing at the wrists. Return to center and lower your hands to your hips. Then lunge to the left.

TOTAL REPETITION: Twelve times for each side.

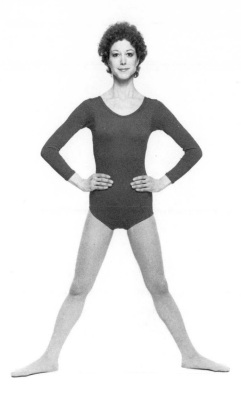

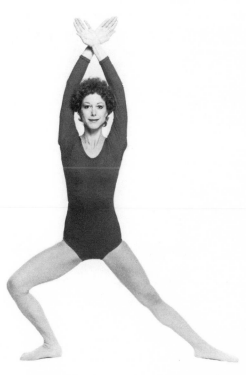

PLACEMENT: Sit with your ankles crossed. Place your hands on your knees.

MOVEMENT: Round your back and lower your head as close to the floor as possible. Simultaneously slide your hands in front of your head. Hold three counts. Uncurl slowly to the original straight-back position.

TOTAL REPETITION: Five times.

Do not let your buttocks lift off of the floor on the forward stretch.

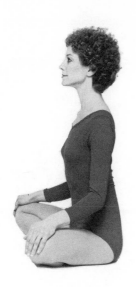

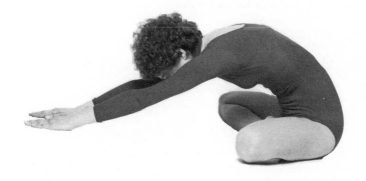

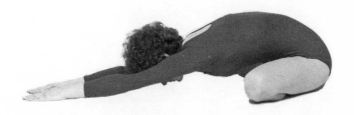

PLACEMENT: Sit with your ankles crossed. Clasp your hands behind your body.

MOVEMENT: Twist to your right. Lower your head and try to touch your left cheek to your right knee. As you lower your head, lift your arms. Hold for two counts. Raise your body and lower your arms before twisting to the left.

TOTAL REPETITION: Five times for each side.

Your buttocks should remain flat on the floor throughout this exercise.

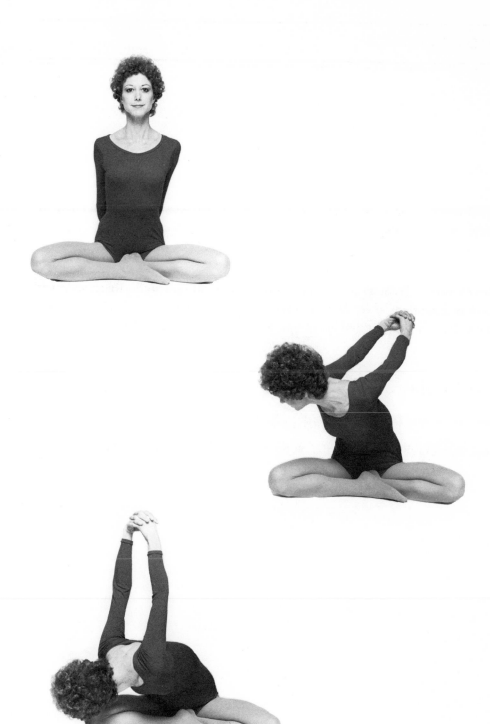

PLACEMENT: Sit down and lean back on your elbows. Bend your knees toward your chest. Place your hands near your hips.

MOVEMENT: Rapidly extend both legs upward fifteen times. Rest for several seconds and repeat.

TOTAL REPETITION: Three times.

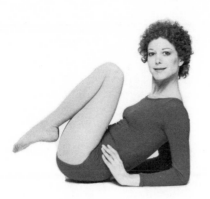

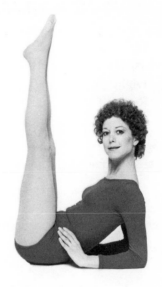

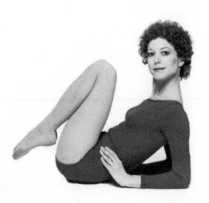

PLACEMENT: Sit down and lean back on your elbows. Place your hands near your waist. Bend your knees close to your chest.

MOVEMENT: Keeping the left knee in place, extend the right leg forward until it is straight. Bring it back into place and extend the left leg. Repeat twenty times. Rest and repeat again.

TOTAL REPETITION: Three times.

Remember to keep your abdominals contracted. This exercise can be done rapidly.

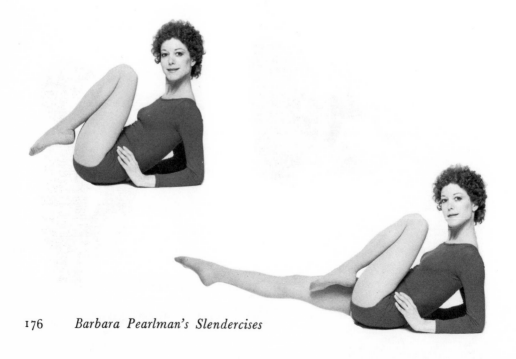

PLACEMENT: Sit with your left leg extended in front. Bend your right knee and clasp your hands around your right ankle. Rest just the toes on the floor.

MOVEMENT: Extend and bend the right leg eight times. Repeat on the left leg.

TOTAL REPETITION: Two times for each leg.

If you are unable to hold your ankle, clasp your hands around your calf instead. Try to extend the leg as high as possible.

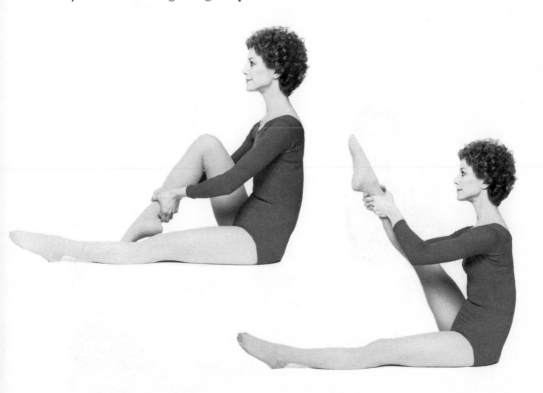

PLACEMENT: Sit with your left leg extended in front. Bend your right knee and clasp your hands around your right ankle. Extend your right leg forward until it is straight.

MOVEMENT: Pull the right leg toward you eight times. Lower the leg and repeat with the left leg.

TOTAL REPETITION: Three times for each leg.

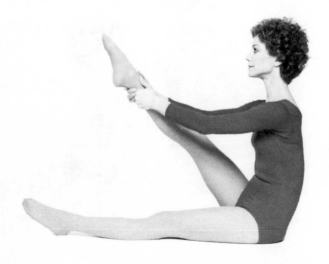

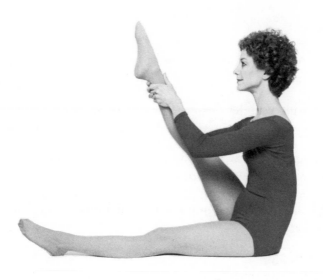

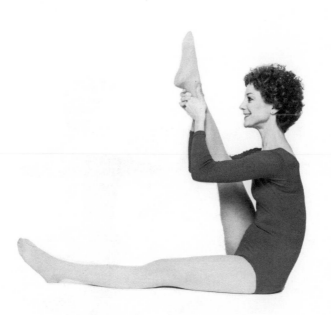

PLACEMENT: Lie on your back, with your knees bent. Place your feet on the floor about twelve inches apart and parallel. Rest your hands on the floor over your head, palms up.

MOVEMENT: Swing your arms forward as you simultaneously lift your upper body off the floor. At the same time straighten your right leg, keeping the foot raised several inches off the floor. Hold two counts, then release to the original position. Repeat with the left leg.

TOTAL REPETITION: Five times for each leg.

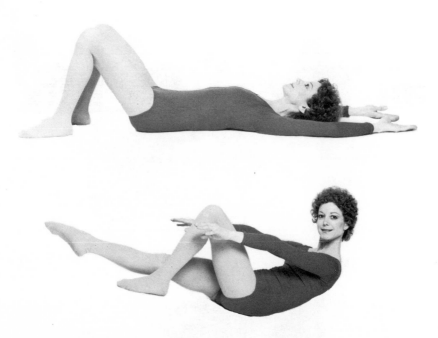

PLACEMENT: Lie on your back with your legs extended upward. Place your arms at your sides.

MOVEMENT: Lower your legs as far to the sides as possible. Bring them together and cross them in a scissorlike motion. Repeat the total movement ten times. Rest and repeat again.

TOTAL REPETITION: Two times.

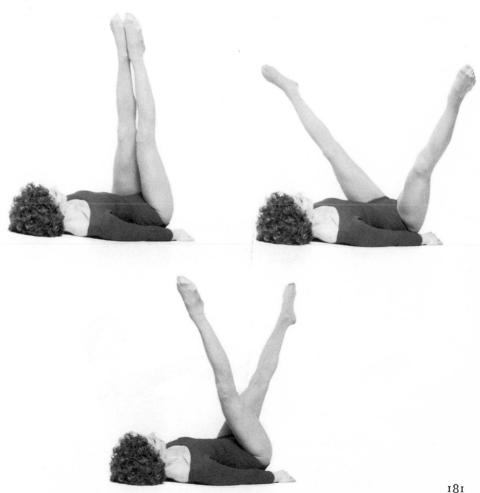